"The brief explanation of Ayurveda, covering seeking balance over imbalance, the stages of various maladies, and a 'Checklist for Health' segues to advice for living one's dharma or life path. Chapters on physical, spiritual, and emotional health, healing wounds from the past, and maintaining healthy relationships, among other subjects, contain guidelines and exercises that, along with recommended resources, make this a comprehensive guide."

— *Booklist*

"Michelle Fondin makes the esoteric and ancient science of Ayurveda accessible to all readers who simply have a desire to improve their health. Her book will introduce you to Ayurveda and supply you with simple, practical, and creative ways to improve every aspect of your health."

— from the foreword by **Sudha Bulusu** and **Dr. Shekhar Annambhotla,** founder of Association of Ayurvedic Professionals of North America

"Includes a comprehensive set of self-assessment questions that allow readers to zero in on their body type's specific needs and best practices for eating plans, addiction treatment, detoxification, and techniques for improving relationships.... *The Wheel of Healing with Ayurveda* brings control and responsibility back to you."

— *New Thought*

CHAKRA HEALING

for

VIBRANT ENERGY

Also by Michelle S. Fondin

The Wheel of Healing with Ayurveda:
An Easy Guide to a Healthy Lifestyle

CHAKRA HEALING
for
VIBRANT ENERGY

Exploring Your 7 Energy
Centers with Mindfulness,
Yoga, and Ayurveda

MICHELLE S. FONDIN

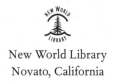

New World Library
Novato, California

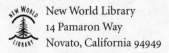

New World Library
14 Pamaron Way
Novato, California 94949

Text design by Tona Pearce Myers

Library of Congress Cataloging-in-Publication Data
Names: Fondin, Michelle S., [date] author.
Title: Chakra healing for vibrant energy : exploring your 7 energy centers
    with mindfulness, yoga, and ayurveda / Michelle S. Fondin.
Description: Novato, California : New World Library, [2018] | Includes
    bibliographical references.
Identifiers: LCCN 2017054223 (print) | LCCN 2018001361 (ebook) |
    ISBN 9781608685356 (Ebook) | ISBN 9781608685349 (alk. paper)
Subjects: LCSH: Mental healing. | Chakras.
Classification: LCC RZ401 (ebook) | LCC RZ401 .F684 2018 (print) |
    DDC 615.8/51—dc23
LC record available at https://lccn.loc.gov/2017054223

First printing, April 2018
ISBN 978-1-60868-534-9
Ebook ISBN 978-1-60868-535-6

Printed in Canada on 100% postconsumer-waste recycled paper

New World Library is proud to be a Gold Certified Environmentally Responsible Publisher. Publisher certification awarded by Green Press Initiative. www.greenpressinitiative.org

10   9   8   7   6   5   4   3   2   1

*This book is dedicated to the loving memory of two of my greatest
teachers of all time, Dr. Wayne W. Dyer and Dr. David Simon.
I felt you were both with me as I wrote these pages.*

*I also dedicate this book to all my teachers who taught me
throughout the years at the Chopra Center,
including Dr. Deepak Chopra, Davidji, and Claire Diab.*

CONTENTS

4. The Heart Chakra: Anahata 89

5. The Throat Chakra: Vishuddha 115

6. The Third-Eye Chakra: Ajna 141

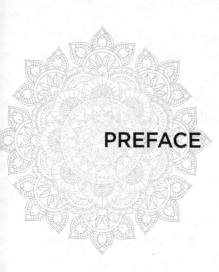

PREFACE

In 1999, at age twenty-eight, I learned I had thyroid cancer. Before this, the word *chakra* had little meaning to me. But suddenly, with this shocking diagnosis, my search for healing rapidly expanded. Perhaps through intuition or past life experience, I had a deep, driving desire to leave no stone unturned when it came to my healing.

I began to search for ways to get to the root cause of why I got cancer in the first place. I knew that if I didn't uproot the disease at its source, I would surely get it again. And in my late twenties, that wasn't an option since I had always planned on living to reach one hundred years old.

In my book *The Wheel of Healing with Ayurveda: An Easy Guide to a Healthy Lifestyle*, I outline the many different discoveries that led to my healing. Allopathic (conventional) medicine played a role, but I intuitively knew that the answers lay in alternative healing modalities. During my exploration, I sat among a pile of library books on alternative medicine and opened up to a life-changing page in Dr. Christiane Northrup's book *Women's Bodies, Women's Wisdom*. The page spoke about the chakras and exploring healing through them. I say it was life-changing because as I was modifying all aspects of my life, an examination of my chakras could now be a focal point for my research into why I got sick.

Changing my diet, increasing my exercise regimen, adding meditation, and improving my relationships all helped in my journey to healing. However, awareness of the chakras gave me an advantage over all other patients suffering from thyroid cancer and other thyroid diseases.

In exploring the thyroid gland and its location in the body, and in learning about the fifth chakra, I started making connections between my current illness and the first twenty-eight years of my life. I looked back and found that most of my illnesses in childhood and young adulthood revolved around the area of the throat. When I was very young I frequently suffered from strep throat or tonsillitis, so much so that doctors repeatedly urged my mother to allow me to have surgery to remove my tonsils. My mother, who was afraid of me going under anesthesia, never agreed to have them taken out.

Then at age seventeen I got mononucleosis. My tonsils were so swollen that they touched in the middle of my throat, closing off my windpipe. I had an abscess in my throat and couldn't breathe. It was so severe that I had to have surgery just so they could open it up to allow me to breathe again.

As I pondered those times with all the throat infections, it became clear to me that something was very wrong and literally blocked in the area of my throat. One of the things the fifth chakra is responsible for is our verbal expression. For me, the illnesses meant exploring why I couldn't properly express myself. I had to ask the questions, "What is holding me back from speaking my truth?" and "Why do I feel I can't speak up?"

I won't go into too much detail, but what I learned was that the circumstances of my upbringing, combined with my being a highly sensitive child, hadn't allowed me the safe space to verbally express myself. In adulthood I had to learn this skill. I believe that without learning this important lesson through the chakras, I would not have completely healed. Patterns that seemed to repeat themselves often throughout my life would have continued to reoccur had I not taken heed of my body's wisdom.

Spiritual and energetic in nature, chakra healing can be a wonderful addition to help you understand the intricacies of your health, just as it did for me. In chronic or advanced stages of a disease, chakra healing can help you hasten your recovery by unblocking the areas of the body that are ailing.

Unlike believing in Santa Claus or the Tooth Fairy, you don't need to wholeheartedly embrace the belief of the chakras to reap the benefits of a chakra healing practice. Belief certainly helps and will probably get you deeper into removal of blockages, but awareness can work just the same. Many things that we don't see — feelings, emotions, thoughts, cellphone connections, air — are real. The following true story from my spiritual journey with alternative health illustrates this point.

In 2005, I was struck with what seemed like either a killer virus or a kidney infection. I had a high fever, my body ached, and I felt sharp, stabbing pains in my kidneys. I summoned all the energy I had just to drive myself to the doctor's office. After I explained my symptoms to the doctor, they took a panel of blood work. I was so weak that they left me to sleep in the examining room for about thirty minutes, and then sent me home. Minutes after I arrived at home, the doctor called me with my blood results. He said he was calling Fairfax Hospital and that I was to go to its emergency room immediately. He told me that my liver enzymes were so high that he feared I had some sort of severe hepatitis. Puzzled and still in extreme pain, I had my husband drive me to the emergency room.

It was a Friday night and the emergency room was extremely crowded, so I had to wait, with my fever and back pains. Not too keen on the possibility that I might have some liver disease, I decided to sit and meditate on my liver and its healing. I waited and meditated, waited and meditated, waited and meditated. For about three hours I visualized my liver with happy faces (you know those yellow emoji smiley faces?) on each cell. I visualized all my liver cells being healthy, happy, and whole. In my mind, there was nothing else I could do. When the staff finally called me in, after they saw my blood results from earlier in the day they put me on an IV immediately. I'm not sure what they were planning, but they were getting ready to perform some kind of medical intervention. However, before taking action they decided to test my blood once more. The results showed that my liver enzymes were back to a normal level. They removed the IV and sent me home. Even more stunning was that my fever and pain were gone, and I felt fine.

Did I spontaneously heal myself through my directed thoughts? I believe I did. Is it possible that something non-physical, such as meditation and visualization, changed the physical? Again, I believe it had everything to do with my healing that day. Is it possible that the blood work was wrong and that the lab mixed up my blood with someone else's? It's possible but not probable. My doctor was just as baffled as I was. He saw what he saw in the labs. He saw how sick I was with acute symptoms. Yet I walked out of the hospital that day without a single symptom and with my blood just as clean as if I had never been sick.

It is my wish that you are able to embrace this very powerful way of healing. The chakras have a magical quality to them. When you begin to read about them and learn about each one, you will feel yourself getting healthier. I wish you a magical journey, my friend. Namasté.

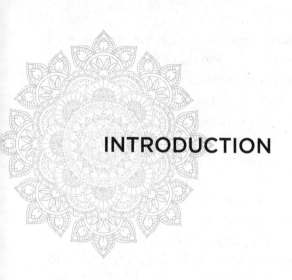

INTRODUCTION

Delving into the world of the chakras is like learning a new language. In a sense, you are. You will be learning many new words in Sanskrit, the ancient language of India. But you will also be immersing yourself in a whole philosophy. In this introduction, all the new terminology might seem overwhelming, but rest assured, the concepts will be explained in great detail throughout the book. Also, you can always turn to the glossary in the back of the book to find out what a term means.

What Is a Chakra?

Chakras are energy centers within the body. The word *chakra* means "wheel" or "disk." Think of the chakras as spinning vortices of energy. Everything is composed of energy and information. Every object emanates from movement and vibration.

The seven main chakras align along the spine, starting at the base of the spine and moving up to the crown of the head.

In the ancient Indian texts called the Vedas, we learn that the physical body is made up of the five great elements called the *mahabhutas*. Those five elements are space (*akasha*), air (*vayu*), water (*jala*), fire (*tejas*), and earth (*prithivi*). The elements are the building blocks of nature and therefore build our bodies as well.

Ancient texts go on to explain that we also have a subtle body. This subtle body is nonphysical and energetic in nature. The subtle body is governed by *prana*, or vital life force. Prana circulates throughout the body and mind. It is responsible for the flow of energy and information. In the subtle body, prana travels through channels called *nadis*. Nadis are circulatory channels within the body such as veins, arteries, the respiratory system, the nervous system, the digestive system, the excretory system, and the reproductive system. Think of nadis as the information highway to your mind, body, soul, and spirit, just as the internet is the information highway that brings information to your browser.

If you have a difficult time grasping the concept of the subtle body, reflect on your mind and thoughts. Thoughts are nonphysical entities. Yet ask anyone who thinks (and that would include all of us), and they will tell you that thoughts are quite real. Scientists have been able to pinpoint areas in the brain where thoughts originate or take place, but slice open a human head and you won't find one thought in there. According to Vedic texts, the mind, intellect, and ego also reside within the subtle body.

Now let's go back to the example of the internet. When you want information, you want it fast, right? You're doing research for a work project or a school report, or getting the scoop on a guy you want to date, and you don't want to wait forever. In the infancy of the internet, with dial-up modems, you could log on, go get a cup of coffee, use the restroom, do your nails, and then the AOL voice of "You've got mail" would finally vibrate in your ever-so-waiting ears. But today, in the world of fiber-optic cables and Wi-Fi, information comes pretty much as quickly as you can type in your question. And when it doesn't come that fast you get frustrated.

For your body to work at an optimal level, the channels through which information travels must be open for that information to get quickly to its destination. If they're blocked, or if there is an abnormality where the information pools in a given area, you won't receive the information you need when you need it. So the nadis are the highways or the fiber-optic cables, and prana is the package of information that needs to be carried.

In total, we have around 88,000 chakras in the body, and the seven main chakras are the information hubs. They gather information on certain aspects of your body, mind, spirit, health, and life. When adequate energy flows to these chakras, that energy fills the area with the information each chakra needs to perform its unique specialty.

Like a highway, your body is constantly moving, changing, growing, and being modified by outside influences. While you may intend to keep the energy and information flowing throughout your body at all times, your lifestyle choices, life experiences, and outside influences may hinder the flow. Fortunately, certain practices can help keep these channels open and information flowing freely, and in this book you will learn what you need to do to achieve this goal quickly and easily.

The Philosophy of the Chakras

The concept of the chakras comes from ancient Indian texts of the Tantric tradition. Tantra is a complicated and important nonreligious philosophy. The Tantric texts are separate from the famously known Indian texts, the Vedas, from whence Ayurveda came.

In the West we tend to associate the word *Tantra* with sex. While sex is mentioned in the Tantric texts, it's meant to be reserved as a practice for only the most advanced yoga practitioners. The main goal of Tantra is to explore the deep mysteries of life and to become liberated within the confines of this world.

The word *Tantra* means "to weave." Tantra is the process of weaving together the body, which has great wisdom, and the mind, which has immense power. By heeding the wisdom of the body and by harnessing the power of the mind you can find the enormous beauty in life on this planet and achieve self-mastery.

The symbolism and stories of the chakras, including their deities and mysticism, are beautiful, colorful, complex, and certainly worth exploring. For the sake of brevity, I will teach you the basics of the chakra system. The foreign words I present come from Sanskrit. For the most part, Sanskrit is no longer spoken but is rich in the roots of language, as many modern English words stem from Sanskrit root words.

The Marriage of Tantra, Ayurveda, and the Yoga Sutras

In order to cognitively grasp the journey into the chakras, it's important to understand a little about the story behind them. According to the Upanishads, a collection of ancient Hindu texts, *purusha* (spirit) is pure universal consciousness. Purusha is formless and unchanging. Out of purusha, *prakruti*, or physical matter, is formed. Prakruti is subject to change and influenced by cause and effect. Everything is a creation of purusha: sun, moon, stars, planets, trees, animals, and humans. Therefore every living thing contains the very essence of the Creator. In a sense, this philosophy isn't much different from the Judeo-Christian view of God expressed in Genesis 2:7: "and breathed into his nostrils the breath of life, and the man became a living being."

According to the Yoga Sutras of Patanjali, the foundational text of yoga philosophy, the main goal in our lifetime is to find our way back to self-realization. The word *self* in the act of self-realization does not refer to our individual selves with our unique personalities and individual bodies but rather the awakening to the Self with a capital *S*, the one from which we originate.

We're born into this world with these bodies, seemingly disconnected from our Creator, so how do we manage?

The second-century sage Patanjali explains in the Yoga Sutras that we have to deal with the three psychic forces of the mind called the *gunas*, which govern the subconscious of all prakruti. The three gunas are *sattva*, *rajas*, and *tamas*.

Sattva is balanced, pure, peaceful, alert, clear-minded, and filled with light.

Rajas is the moving, active energy that is ever-changing.

Tamas is inertia, decay, heaviness, dullness, darkness, and obstruction.

These three qualities of prakruti are necessary in our lives at different times. For example, your spiritual practice is sattvic, and there is a time and place for it in your day. When you need to work and accomplish your goals, you need rajasic energy. When you need to sleep at night, you need tamas so you can get your rest.

In addition to the three gunas, Ayurveda teaches that we have three mind-body types, or *doshas*, which manifest out of the five great elements. The three doshas are Vata (space and air), Pitta (fire and water), and Kapha (water and earth). Each of us has our own unique makeup of the three doshas, which creates our strengths and challenges.

Through the knowledge of the three gunas and the three doshas, we can begin to navigate our body, mind, and life here on earth and start to move toward self-realization.

Since the chakras are part of our physical and subtle bodies, they're also influenced by the gunas and the doshas. The first end goal in the pursuit of self-realization is to live a balanced life. As Tantra teaches, our goal is not to deny the body and the physical realm but to embrace it fully and draw everything good out of it that we possibly can while working our way toward an enlightened state of being, which yoga philosophy refers to as *moksha*, or liberation.

When you're no longer bound by the confines of the gunas and the vacillating and changing nature of the doshas, and you can move through the chakras openly and seamlessly, you have reached enlightenment.

Imagine what it would be like to be in love with every aspect of what it means to be human. True liberation is when love emanates from your being at all times. You're awakened to the gift of each moment and in love with every one. Nothing is a burden, for everything is light, love, and infinite being. You don't need to be anywhere or do anything; this awareness is always with you. For you are it and it is you. That is what we're all here to achieve.

Awakening Kundalini Energy

According to Tantric texts, we have around 72,000 nadis, or circulatory channels, in the body, which transport prana. In our study of the chakras, we will focus only on the Shushumna nadi, the Ida nadi, and the Pingala nadi. The Shushumna nadi is the energy channel that starts at the base of the spine in the area of the first chakra. It's where the Kundalini Shakti (creative energy) sits like a serpent, coiled up in three rings, waiting to spring forth into action and wake up the chakras. The Shushumna nadi travels up the length of the spine in a channel behind the spinal cord to the crown of the head at the seventh chakra. From the base of the Shushumna nadi arise two other nadis, the Ida nadi and the Pingala nadi. The Ida nadi is lunar in nature: passive, gentle, and feminine. The Pingala nadi is solar: warm, stimulating, and masculine. The Ida nadi starts and ends on the left side of the Shushumna nadi, and the Pingala nadi starts and ends on the right side. The Ida and Pingala nadis cross at every chakra, and all three of these nadis meet at the sixth, or third-eye, chakra. In our bodies the Ida and Pingala nadis alternate in dominance. Generally the Ida nadi dominates the right side of the brain, and the Pingala dominates the left side.

Kundalini energy is awakened through purification of the body and mind. There are many practices to cleanse the physical body, including eating a clean diet; abstaining from impure substances; detoxifying through Ayurvedic daily practices such as tongue scraping and nasal washing with a neti pot and *nasya* (infused oil); and the Ayurvedic seasonal cleansing practices of *panchakarma*, or five actions. In addition, one must practice yoga *asanas* (physical postures, what we in the West generally think of as "yoga") and *pranayama* (breathing techniques).

Purifying the mind comes with the practice of the eight limbs of yoga: the *yamas, niyamas, asana, pranayama, pratyahara, darana, dhyana,* and *samadhi.*

In the following chapters I will describe many of these techniques as they pertain to each chakra.

Understanding the Dual Nature of the Chakras — and of Life Itself

In this world of duality, where everything has its opposite, we must strive to understand both sides. It can be destructive to have only light without darkness, only wakefulness with no sleep, and only full bellies with no hunger. Through our trials and tribulations on our earthly journey, we seek to enhance the pleasurable and try to minimize the unpleasant. However, living a balanced life is about recognizing both sides. As you look back at your past, you may notice that unexpected beauty erupted and developed in your moments of strife and anguish. For example, you may have met your husband when you had a flat tire and he offered to change it for you. Or maybe you overcame an addiction and are now helping others overcome addictions and live sober and clean lives.

Often when we're on a spiritual journey, we want the outcome of enlightenment and spiritual connection without understanding where we came from. You were born into the physical realm through your earthly mother. You chose this incarnation, and there is nothing wrong with it. When you signed up to come here, you promised to fulfill certain duties, called *dharma*, and take on certain responsibilities. Unless you fully embrace the dualistic nature of your existence in this life, you will continue to have a difficult time reaching the spiritual heights you seek.

In every chakra, as in life, there are two possible states: a balanced state and an excessive or depleted state, which indicates an imbalance. As we have learned through life's lessons, too much or too little of anything can be destructive and unhealthy. You may have heard the expression "Money is the root of all evil." The expression implies that having too much money and hoarding it can be detrimental. And too little money, which leads to lack, poverty, theft, hunger, and depression, can also be ruinous. Both extremes can lead to a life you don't desire.

I received a reading from an astrologer friend last fall. He had an interesting and truthful perspective I had never heard before in an astrology reading. In my astrological chart I have an unfavorable aspect from the planet Saturn, which is omnipresent in my life. If you know anything about astrology, no one wants Saturn to show up all the time and interfere in their life. Saturn is a huge, slow-moving planet that can create delays, reduce potential, and be a huge obstacle in accomplishing things. As my friend explained, Saturn also has rings, which are binding. He gave the example of a wedding ring. He explained that a wedding band symbolically binds you to the other person and puts a certain number of restrictions on your life. So as he gave me this "bad news," I was thinking, *Holy cow! That's why I've had such a hard time getting my career off the ground.* But at that moment he gave me another perspective, the opposite side of a Saturn aspect.

He explained that while Saturn creates obstacles and delays, it also has a positive side to it. For example, a Saturn aspect can make you humble and inclined to show humility to others and not be boastful. Saturn can make a person hunker down and get things done, such as conducting research for a term paper or writing a book. It can give you the discipline to focus on painting a picture or building a house. In other words, he displayed the beauty of a Saturn aspect to me.

Then he taught me how to work with Saturn versus fighting against it. He suggested that when I see Saturn arrive with its delays, closed doors, and seemingly immovable boulders, I should welcome it in, offer it a cup of tea, and thank it for its wisdom. He offered me the wisdom that the more I accept Saturn as a part of my life, the more Saturn will offer me its gifts. As a result of my acceptance, I was able to change my perspective on a force I thought had been ruining my life. It's now a force of strength for me.

The chakras — especially the first three, which are the chakras of matter — work in the same way. Oftentimes when we're presented with the aspects of the chakras, we see only the imbalances or challenging sides to them. We want to rush through the first three and skip ahead to the more spiritual chakras. It's important to remember the blessings in each chakra, even when we struggle with them. The power comes in embracing them and bringing awareness to their beauty. What we consider to be the ugliness of human existence is also what brings us joy.

This reminds me of an old saying I once read: "Laughter is like changing a baby's diaper; it doesn't solve anything, but it sure improves the situation." If you have ever changed a baby's diaper, you know this. The act of wiping the baby clean, applying some lotion, and putting on a clean diaper is part of this sometimes smelly human existence. On top of it, you know that in a few hours you're going to have to do it all over again. But boy, doesn't that baby smell marvelous? And you have great memories of hugging, snuggling, and enjoying your baby during this mundane and kind of gross experience. That is duality.

Reasons the Chakras Might Get Blocked

A blocked chakra means energy is stuck or hindered. You might think of it as a blocked artery. In order for energy and information to flow, the channels through which they flow must be open. You will have difficulty getting to work on time if the roads are blocked by traffic. In the same way, the chakras cannot work at optimal levels when the pathways have blockages. These blockages can be physical, emotional or psychological, spiritual, karmic, or energetic.

The blocks can be physical, in the literal sense, such as fatty deposits in the arteries, a tumor, a cyst, or excess waste. We can create blockages in the physical body through poor dietary choices, lack of exercise, overexertion, and lifestyle choices such as overwork, drug use, or lack of sleep.

Blocks in the chakras can also be emotional or psychological, such as stored emotions from the past or mental illness such as anxiety, depression, or addiction. We accumulate emotional toxins and residue from not properly processing and digesting emotions and experiences. These toxins result in blocking the energy flow of the chakras.

Blocks can be spiritual in nature. They can come from outside spiritual forces or from within. If we refuse to honor the spiritual side of who we are, we block the higher chakras. Being spiritually rigid and strict can also restrict the flow of energy. Remember, whether the forces are external or internal, without your conscious awareness they can create harm.

Blockages can also come from our karma. The word *karma* in Sanskrit literally means "action." In life we perform actions that are good or nourishing, bad or harmful, or neutral. An example of a good action might be giving money to charity. A bad action might be intentionally lying or deceiving. A neutral action might be making the bed (which, if you dig deeper, can also be considered a good action, depending on the circumstances). In the East, certain religions and philosophies adhere to the principle that we accumulate karma throughout lifetimes, and we carry it forth into our current life. The definition of karma, in this sense, assumes a belief in reincarnation and asserts that karma is not simply the action performed but also the consequences of that action. Good karma carried forward can give us favor in our current lifetime. Bad karma is a debt we must repay in this or future lifetimes.

Whether or not you believe in reincarnation or the explanation of karma, you can learn to appreciate and grasp the concept. Have you ever heard anyone say that they constantly suffer from bad luck? The bad luck may be more about paying back a karmic debt of which they aren't even aware. You've surely heard the adages "What goes around comes around" and "You reap what you sow." These expressions explain the essence of karma. Often, in our minds, karma has negative connotations. But note that you can accumulate good karma through good actions or service to others.

Finally, the blocks can be energetic. I explained a little about energetic blockages when I spoke about my astrological chart. We are a part of this earth, our solar system, and the universe. The influence of the earth's energy and elements, as well as of the energy of the sun, moon, and planets in our solar system, is strong and undeniable. Ayurveda, the five-thousand-year-old medical system from India, recognizes these energetic forces and acknowledges them as a means of healing. You can learn more about Ayurveda by reading my book *The Wheel of Healing with Ayurveda: An Easy Guide to a Healthy Lifestyle.* Ayurveda works on the principles of the five elements — space, air, fire, water, and earth — which work together to create the three doshas, or mind-body types, of Vata (space and air), Pitta (fire and water), and Kapha (water and earth). These elements and mind-body types are relevant in recognizing energetic blocks within your body and the chakras. This awareness will give you more tools toward your healing of the chakras and provide a superspeed highway to creating energy flow.

Awareness

In any spiritual practice, awareness is the first key to awakening. When you come out of a holiday, realize that you can't fit into your jeans, and get on the scale, you become aware that you may need to lose weight. Without this awareness, you will do nothing to change. Awareness means coming out of the dark and stepping into the light. Most often awareness is for our greater good at the time it's revealed to us. Yet we are sometimes afraid of what we might find. Awakening can mean we find ourselves in a place where we don't want to be. Awareness can mean we now see the mess we must clean up. Sometimes our friend awareness comes as a slap on the face that doesn't feel too good. Then our friend denial comes in and coaxes us back to what feels good but may not be right.

You are human. You have a physical body, an emotional body, and an energetic body. You are also a spirit with a spiritual existence that is currently bound by a body. Awakening can come only when we accept the entire package. Yet our other friend, the mind, also comes in and tries to convince us that one way is better than another. For example, the mind tries to say, "If only you had better parents, you might be in a better financial situation." Then the ego comes along and adds its two cents: "Yeah, and if your boss treated you better, you might have gotten that raise you deserve." So all these parts create who you are, and balance comes from accepting every part.

As you work through the chakras, things will come up. Grievances, hurt, past afflictions, and present discomforts will arise and make themselves known to you. This is a good thing and what you want for healing. You certainly don't have to accept them right away. Just make yourself aware of them. Notice them. Say hello. Watch them as you would a movie on a screen. Sometimes awareness alone will heal that which ails you.

Balancing Your Chakras

Your exploration of healing through the chakras can add a layer of beauty and depth to your health and well-being. Imagine choosing a wedding cake. You could probably get by with a yellow cake and white frosting. But the beauty comes in when a pastry chef infuses chocolate ganache into the center, layers the cake in creative ways, and adds intricate decorations to each layer and an eye-popping topper. You then have a work of art to display at your wedding rather than a plain single-layer cake. The intricacy of that wedding cake mirrors the depth of layers in a marriage and the magic of its beginning at the wedding celebration.

The layers of your health are no different. You can focus on the physical body and have allopathic or Western medicine fix it when something goes wrong. Or you can focus on preventive health through diet, exercise, yoga, meditation, and other healing practices such as emotional and spiritual healing.

I will give you tools to balance the seven main chakras, with one chapter devoted to each chakra. For each of the chakras I provide descriptions of pranayama (breathing) techniques and yoga poses. You can check out demonstrations of all of these on my YouTube channel: www.youtube.com/c/Michelle FondinAuthor. While healing your chakras, practice these poses once in the morning and once in the evening. I have also included dietary recommendations, a guided meditation, thoughts to ponder for the day, and other areas to explore for emotional and spiritual healing, with practices such as prayer, visualization, and chanting. I also offer suggestions for taking your energetic healing a step further through work with colors and gems: you can wear the color of the chakra you're healing, and carry with you throughout your day the crystal or gem associated with that chakra.

Through these practices you can heal your chakras in seven days. You can repeat these seven days every week for a year, going deeper into your awareness and healing each week. Or you can take seven months and dedicate your practice to one chakra for each month. Or you can go at your own pace, spending more time on certain chakras than others, as needed. There is no single best way to go about this healing practice. I know that many of you are good, disciplined students and will try to do every single suggestion in each chapter. Instead of attempting to do everything in one day, see which healing practices call to you most, and try those first. If you let it, your intuition will guide the way.

As with the practice of yoga asanas, you don't need to adhere to any particular religion, sect, or spiritual belief to heal with the chakras. You only need to be open to your body's inner wisdom and the energy field that surrounds you. Now is the moment you might ask, "How do I tune in to my energy field?" The answer is, you are already tuned in to your energy field.

Have you ever walked into a room filled with tension and felt that the air was so thick you could cut it with a knife? Or have you felt a rush of energy when walking into a sports stadium or rock concert? You're perceiving energy all the time, but you're not often aware that you're aware.

Expanding your perception is something that happens naturally as a result of spiritual practice. As you go through life on this physical plane, you get accustomed to a narrow vision, seeing only things that are in your pathway. We all do this, as it's a way our brains filter out the "noise" to get us through our days without getting distracted all the time. However, it's not so useful when it comes to your health and well-being. A broadened perspective is an asset and will allow you to notice subtle changes in your body.

Body awareness, mindfulness, and learning how to direct your thoughts are ways in which you can start to attain better health. Working with your chakra energy can help you with early detection before an illness becomes full-blown, or it can help in your healing in the midst of a disease, as it did in my case.

Finally, it can be helpful to look at the ailments associated with each of the chakras. When I was ill with thyroid cancer, my healing ultimately took place when I took a good look at the fifth chakra. I believe all diseases are messages from the body indicating that something is off. In looking at diseases you might be experiencing, you can take a deeper look by knowing which chakra is out of balance. Taking medicine or removing a tumor or even an organ or body part might be necessary to stop the spread of the disease, but it won't help you get to the root of it. Considering the "why" is important to achieve complete and total healing. Sometimes you don't get an answer. But often you do. Through chakra balancing you learn to listen to your intuition, that still, small voice inside you, and it will give you an inner knowing of how to heal.

1 THE ROOT CHAKRA
Muladhara

ELEMENT: Earth (Prithivi)
COLOR: Red
MANTRA SOUND: *LAM*

Our journey begins at the base of the spine with the first chakra, Muladhara. The word *Muladhara* means "foundation" or "base" and comes from the two Sanskrit words *mul*, meaning "base," and *adhara*, meaning "support" or "foundation." This is the first of the three elemental or material chakras in the body, and it's the thickest and densest chakra of the seven. While it's associated with our being in our most basic state, it's no less important than the other chakras on our journey. In fact, it's the primary and fundamental chakra we must balance in order to enjoy our time here on earth.

The element of Muladhara is earth, or *prithivi* in Sanskrit. We are bound to earth through gravity. Everything we do to remain on earth is found here. Think of the word *survival*. We must find shelter, eat, sleep, and procreate. We must protect our environment, including nature and Mother Earth. We must find jobs, do work, and make money to fulfill our needs. We must obey the laws of nature, our environment, and society.

In the body, the first chakra is located in the middle of the perineum and includes the coccyx (tailbone), the pelvis, the base of the spine, and the first three vertebrae. The sense associated with the first chakra is smell, and the sense organ is the nose.

The color we attribute to the base chakra is deep red. The mantra, or *bija* (seed) sound, we vocalize for the first chakra is *LAM*.

First Chakra Ailments

While the earth element rules the first chakra, the ailments that occur with its imbalance resemble the same diseases or imbalances that occur with the Ayurvedic mind-body type Vata, which is governed not by earth but by space and air. As you may deduct, the elements of space and air are polar opposites of the element earth. Therefore, healing can begin when you bring balance back to the earth element through proper grounding to counteract the excessive space and air.

First-chakra blockages may include constipation, hemorrhoids, sciatica pain, degenerative arthritis, knee troubles, obesity, anorexia nervosa or other eating disorders, anxiety disorders, fears, nightmares, and psychosis. Almost all of these symptoms and disorders are directly related to imbalances in the Vata dosha or space and air mind-body type. Obesity would be the only ailment in this list caused by an excessive amount of the Kapha dosha, which is composed of water and earth.

First Chakra Energy: Solid Like a Rock

The energy of the first chakra is vital to our existence. It's a downward energy that grounds us and gives us stability. In the body, first-chakra energy governs bone structure, feet, legs, and the large intestine to digest food. Everything we eat comes from the earth and its energy. The homes we build and the structures we enjoy, such as libraries, movie theaters, and skyscrapers, all come from first chakra energy. Gravity keeps us in communion with our planet. The art of manifesting emanates from acceptance of our material existence.

Tamas is the type of energy that rules Muladhara. Tamasic energy is slow, dull, inert. The Ayurvedic dosha that dominates the first chakra is Kapha, which is comprised of the elements of water and earth.

An overabundance of tamasic energy can make a person sluggish, lazy, overweight, and complacent. However, tamas is necessary when a pregnant woman grows a baby. She needs to be grounded, slow down, take more naps, reduce her activities, and eat more food. The same goes for the seasons. Winter is a tamasic season when nothing appears to be going on and nature seems dormant. Animals hibernate. Grass and trees stop growing. But this period of rest is necessary for the outburst of activity in the spring.

Kapha energy is similar to tamasic energy. A healthy Kapha person is grounded, slow, methodical, humble, and down-to-earth. Babies go through a Kapha phase to be able to experience life on earth fully and to grow properly. The two sense organs of Kapha are the nose and mouth (tongue: taste). All babies first experience the world by putting things in their mouths. Babies sleep more than older children and adults. They are drawn to and fascinated by nature and the earth's elements. They are thus perfect expressions of fully embracing earth energy.

Adult Kapha types who are living in balance are peaceful people to be around. They are loving, affectionate, and kind.

Their solid foundation gives comfort to others by being the stable pillars to lean on.

Our Societal Relationship with the Earth Element

While we must embrace earth energy to grow, expand, and raise our levels of consciousness, modern society tends to move us in the opposite direction of where we need to go.

Our experience of being on earth and staying grounded requires us to have direct contact with the material. In other words, when we take walks in nature, have picnics on the beach, gather with others for dinner or conversation, and take care of animals, we are directly interacting with the energy that grounds us. Many of our experiences today happen virtually. We are living in the ether without having a solid foundation. While being on our smartphones, computers, and tablets involves touching something material, we engage in a virtual reality through such technology. We talk or text with people out there in any number of places. We play games with people or bots without knowing the difference. We have one-sided conversations as we post on social media, hoping that someone will respond. These experiences keep us ungrounded. In addition, we live in a society that likes to take pills, drugs, and alcohol to transform our state. We seek the transformative ecstasy of spirit without having the proper roots.

As a result, we eat a lot of food to try to ground ourselves. Because the body has an innate intelligence, it tells us we need to do something to bring ourselves down to earth. So we consume loads of calories seeking the grounded, comforting feelings of a loving mother's warm embrace. Yet too much food and eating the wrong foods does the opposite of making us feel grounded and safe. It disconnects us from the body and our true needs and desires.

In order to experience the earth, you must get back to it. Relearn how to enjoy life without a device in front of your eyes, in your ears, or in your pocket. Meet people face-to-face. Take walks and listen to the sounds of nature. Cook foods from scratch. Let the sunshine penetrate your face. Gaze at the stars. Get comfortable being here rather than somewhere else. Make earth your home again.

Living Life in the Muladhara Chakra: Security

In each of the chakras, there is a difference between embracing and accepting the energy and gifts from that chakra and living solely from that chakra. As you awaken to the limitations in each chakra, you are driven to discover ways to operate from different levels of consciousness. It's human nature to want to explore and grow. However, not everyone operates from this level of thinking. Many people accept limitations as hard boundaries and don't seek to move beyond them. If you're ready to extend beyond the limitations of your chakras, it's important to understand what living at the level of each chakra looks like.

People who live in first-chakra energy are in survival mode. Their basic emotion is fear. They are only concerned with security and how to obtain it. The parts of the brain responsible for survival are the brain stem, or medulla, and the limbic system, comprised of the amygdala and the hippocampus. Fight-or-flight is a primitive response hardwired in these parts of the brain, a reaction to fear and a need for survival. In animals, the onset of this primitive response helps them determine if they will fight predators or run away. Fight-or-flight is a chain reaction that begins in the amygdala. It includes a release of stress hormones, such as cortisol, adrenaline, and noradrenaline. Your heart races, your blood pressure goes up, your blood platelets get sticky, your immune system becomes suppressed, your blood is shunted away from your digestive organs and moved toward the limbs; you sweat and feel compelled to either run or fight.

This primitive response to real and present danger is useful sometimes. Let's suppose your small child runs into the street after a ball. You must have quick energy to run after him to save him from a moving car. Or if you're driving and another vehicle suddenly pulls out in front of you, you need fight-or-flight to slam on the brakes. However, the fight-or-flight response isn't so useful when your life isn't in danger and you're responding to fear rather than reality. People who live solely from the first chakra respond to fear most of the time. Their motives are fear of lack, fear of loss, fear of not enough, and the "what if…?" syndrome.

First chakra people would rather stay in a dissatisfying job than risk losing job security or a steady paycheck. They are not often leaders but followers with blind obedience. They fear standing out from the crowd and would rather blend in.

The need to fight for security can be seen in first chakra people's job choices. They might choose to be soldiers or police officers to ensure security of their cities or countries. They constantly seek favor and acceptance from their superiors and work hard to serve them. First chakra people strive for rewards while greatly fearing punishment. While they obey and look up to authority, they are often harsh with people under them.

A person living from an instinctive and primal response is like a small child. Without proper instruction and limitations, a child can become greedy or hoard material goods. She can refrain from sharing. She can lash out physically at another child if she's dissatisfied or hurt, or doesn't get her way. She can ignore proper etiquette or societal norms. She can lose her temper and say mean things out of anger.

While all of us can and do revert back to this type of behavior some of the time, a first chakra person lives this way most of the time.

Trust is a big issue for first chakra people. We learn trust in the first two years of life through the care of our parents and caretakers. If the care is consistent, loving, and present, we develop trust in others and in our environment. Through trust we develop the value of hope. However, if we're in a home where a parent is absent, or our needs are delayed or not taken care of properly, we learn to distrust that others or our environment will provide for us. Those stuck in the first chakra seem to be constantly working out trust issues, which is why they're fearful.

Recognizing First Chakra Imbalances

The first way to move beyond a limitation is to recognize it. As I pointed out, each object and concept in life has its strengths and weaknesses. That is the nature of duality. The Muladhara chakra keeps us rooted to the earth. It allows us to fully enjoy our earthly existence and manifest our desires into material objects. Muladhara is solid, thick, dense, and real.

The flip side of Muladhara is excessive fear that leads to worry, anxiety, and lack of trust. You can feel the weight of the gravitational pull downward and feel burdened and heavy. In an effort to ground yourself, you can overeat, which leads to being overweight or obese and feeling disconnected from your body.

People with shaky foundations may feel that they never have enough or that what they do have will be taken away. They might hoard material goods and pile them up in their homes. They can be stingy or miserly with their money.

Think of the principle of survival of the fittest. When we are stuck in the first chakra, this becomes our guiding principle.

Accepting First Chakra Gifts

We live on this beautiful, bountiful planet called Earth. Our planet is filled with lavish abundance. Our ability to experience this planet through our senses is what can make us appreciate the objects that this life has to offer. First chakra gifts tell us we're not in lack. All we have to do is look around and see the plentiful resources at our disposal. Nature brings us these gifts we don't have to pay for. There is enough for everyone.

While gravity can seem weighty, it's necessary for us to live out our purpose in life. We need to dig our hands into the dirt (so to speak) and live in the here and now.

Healing Muladhara

> DAILY AFFIRMATION
>
> I am secure and grounded. My
> basic needs are met. I am fearless.

 Healing the Physical Body

Healing in the first chakra comes with accepting that you have a physical body and learning to appreciate and love it. Many people view their bodies as a hindrance to getting where they want to go. They say things like "Oh, eating is such an inconvenience" or "If I didn't have to go to the bathroom or sleep so much, I could get more done." Societal norms have us believe that the body is designed to break down, experience disease, and get worse with age. This is simply not true. Those are just beliefs.

Women often have body image issues. They feel shameful

or hate their bodies. They want their breasts to be smaller or bigger. They feel their thighs are too fat or their bottom is too thin. Conversely, men can sometimes ignore the needs of their bodies by forgetting to get a checkup or not paying closer attention to the early physical signs of disease.

I recently had an Ayurvedic consultation with a client who has an inflammatory autoimmune disease. She was worried about taking prednisone daily and wanted to get off it, but every time she tried, she experienced the pain of her disease. In our consultation I discovered that her primary dosha was Vata and she was only eating once a day and was barely sleeping. I explained to her that if she wanted her body to heal, she had to get back into her body. She's a highly creative individual and loves her creative work. She embraces her space and air qualities so much that she lives daily in the ether and reinforces that by not eating or sleeping. Getting back into her body means she needs to take care of it and do grounding practices. Then, and only then, will she be able to heal from her autoimmune disease.

Your beautiful body is comprised of the elements of the earth: space, air, fire, water, and earth. You're a part of this amazing and miraculous existence. First, accepting your body as a vehicle through which you experience life is essential. Second, honoring your body by feeding it the proper foods, exercising it, and giving it adequate sleep shows that you respect it.

Eating as a Sacred Act

In Western society we don't take time to appreciate the food we eat daily. We often eat food on the go, in our vehicles or while walking, or we skip meals throughout the day. Preparing food, serving it, and eating it should be a sacred act. Our body is the only channel through which we enjoy our time on earth. Loving your body means appreciating its needs and benefiting from its strengths.

To reconnect with your body through the act of eating, commit to taking at least one meal each week in silence. Shop for your food in gratitude and excitement at the prospect of sharing the gift of a meal with your body. Prepare the food with love. Take the time to smell your food and taste each and every bite. Be grateful to Mother Earth for providing you with the nourishment and sustenance that you need to live.

PRACTICING BODY ACCEPTANCE

Your body is giving you the gift of life every day. If you can get up and walk, run, jump, and bend, you have so many blessings. I love what Dr. Wayne Dyer used to say: "We should have a liver appreciation day." In other words, celebrate the parts of your body you normally take for granted. When I'm teaching yoga I sometimes have my students massage their own feet and thank their feet for supporting them.

Look at your naked body in a mirror. You read that correctly. Look at it. Send it love and appreciate its beauty.

YOGA ASANAS AND PRANAYAMA EXERCISES TO HEAL THE FIRST CHAKRA

Practicing yoga is a great way to heal your chakras. To heal the first chakra, you will focus on grounding poses or any pose that engages the base of the spine and the area of the perineum.

To view a video demo of these exercises, go to
www.youtube.com/c/MichelleFondinAuthor.
Click on the Playlists tab, and select
Chakra Healing Asanas & Pranayamas.
Scroll down the list until you find the one you're looking for.

Three-Part Breath — *Dirgha***:** Sit comfortably with your eyes closed. As you breathe, inflate your belly like a balloon on the inhalation and deflate the belly on the exhalation. The complete breath is done through the nose only, with the lips closed. Begin the three-part breath by inhaling first from your lower belly, below your belly button, then expanding to the midbelly, and then allowing the air to rise up into your chest. As you exhale, deflate your chest, then your midbelly, and finally your lower abdomen. Practice this breathing technique for three to five minutes. For first chakra balancing, once you get comfortable with this breathing practice, focus on the tip of your nose while practicing the complete version.

Mula Bandha **and Kegels:** The word *bandha* means "lock" or "hold." And, of course, *mula* means "root." So the *mula bandha* is the root lock. If you are a woman and have practiced Kegel exercises, you will find mula bandha is similar in nature. For a Kegel exercise, a woman contracts the muscles in the perineum, holds for several seconds, and repeats the exercise many times. Both men and women can practice mula bandha. For a man, you contract the muscles between the anus and the testes. For a woman, you contract the muscles at the bottom of the pelvic floor. Hold this lock for as long as you can; some yoga practitioners suggest holding it for the entire class.

Mula bandha stimulates the pelvic nerves, the genital system, the endocrine system, and the excretory system. Regular practice of the root lock can relieve constipation and mild depression.

Knee to Chest Pose — *Pavanamuktasana***:** Lie flat on your back. Bring your right knee to your chest while your left leg is still elongated on the floor. Clasp your hands below your right knee. Keep your head on the floor and inflate your belly, allowing it to puff out. On the exhalation, bend your elbows and bring your knee closer to your chest. You're stimulating the ascending and transverse colon, liver, and right kidney. After five to seven breaths, release your right leg to the floor. Bring your left knee to your chest and repeat. On the left side you're stimulating the descending colon, the large intestine, and the left kidney.

Lotus Flexion — *Padmasana*: Sit cross-legged on the floor with your back erect and tall. Place your left foot in to press on the perineum. If you can, place your right foot on top of your left thigh in a half lotus pose. Make sure your sitting bones are rooted down and pressed to the earth. Clasp your hands behind you, interlacing your fingers, and straighten your arms behind your back. Lift the spine tall, then hinge from your hips, and bring your upper body forward toward the floor in front of you. Bring your arms up off your back in the forward bend as much as you can. Hold the pose for five to seven breaths.

Squatting Pose — *Malasana*: Stand with your feet a little wider than hip-width apart and your toes turned slightly out. Sit into a squat as if you were sitting in a chair, but lower your tailbone until it's a few inches from the floor. It's okay if your heels lift up slightly. Place your hands in prayer posture with your elbows gently pushing out on each inner thigh. Lengthen through your spine, lower your shoulders, and lift the crown of your head. You can use a yoga block to sit on in this pose if your hips are tight or the squat is hard on your knees. Practicing Kegels or mula bandha (see description above) is ideal in this pose. If you can, hold this pose for up to one minute.

Pelvic Tilts: Lie flat on your back with your knees bent and your feet flat on the floor, hip-width apart and parallel, with your toes pointing forward. Walk your heels close to your bottom. Place your arms alongside you with your palms facing down. The position looks like a preparation for bridge pose (*setu bandhasana*), a yoga asana you may be familiar with (described on page 130). Begin the tilt by squeezing your buttocks and lifting your tailbone and first three vertebrae, one vertebra at a time. Then squeeze, hold for five seconds, lower, and release. Repeat this exercise twenty-five times. Pelvic tilts bring heat and energy to the first chakra, stimulating all the nerves.

Standing Mountain Pose — *Tadasana*: Stand tall with your feet parallel and toes pointed forward. A great way to do this grounding pose is to use a yoga block and place it between your upper thighs. Spread out your toes, and firmly plant your feet on the floor. Draw the energy up through your legs. Squeeze your buttocks while slightly opening your thighs outward. Stack your vertebrae, each one on top of the one below, and lift the crown of your head with your head in a neutral position. Roll your shoulders back and down, and allow your arms to hang like plumb lines. Close your eyes and feel the dynamic of your feet firmly rooted to the earth and the crown of your head floating upward toward the sky. Notice how good it feels to be balanced, grounded, and immovable.

Balancing the First Chakra through Food

It's important on your healing journey to eat only whole foods that are fresh and come directly from the earth. Reduce your consumption of processed, packaged, canned, or frozen food.

When you're feeling ungrounded, eat heavier foods such as proteins, hearty soups, bread, oils, and sweet fruit. You can also focus on eating root vegetables and potatoes. If you're feeling too heavy and sluggish, try eating what Ayurveda calls a Kapha-pacifying diet: focus on bitter, pungent, and astringent tastes; eat more beans, lentils, leafy green vegetables, and whole grains such as quinoa; reduce meat consumption.

WEIGHT LIFTING TO BALANCE MULADHARA

Those who live mainly focused on the first chakra instinctually build up their muscles through weight training. In fact, lifting weights is an excellent way to physically balance the first chakra. You must be grounded to lift weights; otherwise you would topple over under the weight. The heaviness (even with lighter weights) will make you stronger and more rooted to the earth. Weight training is a great way to play around with gravity, the first chakra energy.

 ## Healing the Emotional and Energetic Body

When it comes to mental and emotional healing in the first chakra, you need to think about three basic thought concepts: worry, trust, and security.

WORRY

We all suffer from worry at one time or another. It's not always easy to delve into the past and think about our development of trust and security, but it might be worth doing this if you struggle with issues of trust or worry. Concern is valid at times, such as when you have difficulty paying bills on time or your marriage is on shaky ground. Yet worry isn't warranted if you can do nothing to change the situation.

In many different religions and spiritual practices we're warned not to worry. In the Bible, Jesus says in Matthew 6:27, "Can all your worries add a single moment to your life?" In all 12-step programs, the meetings conclude with the Serenity Prayer:

> *God, grant me the serenity to accept the things I cannot*
> *   change,*
> *The courage to change the things I can,*
> *And the wisdom to know the difference.*

Worry is a blockage in and of itself. It blocks the flow of energy to creative solutions. Worry causes us to act out of fear instead of love. When we act out of fear — or rather react, in most cases — we usually create new problems and obstacles.

Maybe you developed worry from your upbringing — maybe your parents constantly worried. Or perhaps you developed worry from uncertain circumstances in your past, such as parents divorcing, poverty, or a dysfunctional family home. Whatever the case, you have the power to change it now. You can start by saying the Serenity Prayer to yourself daily and truly thinking about the things you can change versus the things you can't.

TRUST

If you didn't grow up with a healthy sense of trust, you may find it difficult to trust others and your environment. There is no magic bullet to building trust back to a normal level. But if you're open to learning, you can take baby steps toward its attainment. As you think about the concept of trust, think about things in the environment that are certain. For example, you can trust that the sun will rise each morning and set each night. You can trust that you have twenty-four hours in the day. You can trust that there are four seasons and certain celebrations or milestones on the calendar. You can trust that your body will need between six and nine hours of sleep per night, depending on your personal needs. You can trust that you will need to eat about three times per day and that if you follow the principles of healthy living, your body will perform for you.

Think about all the things you already trust but take for granted. For example, do you have a bank account? Do you deposit money into it? If you do, you trust that the bank will eventually give you back the money when you need it. Do you drive a car? If so, you trust all the other drivers to stay in their lanes and not run into you.

When it comes to people and loved ones, first try noticing little things you trust. When a boyfriend shows up on time for a date, you learn to trust him. Or when a new friend remembers it's your birthday, you begin to trust that she cares for you. Do you see how trust is a flowing dynamic? We tend to overlook the little gestures in relationships, even though trust building is usually an accumulation of a lot of little things.

When you approach "feeling" concepts such as trust from the perspective of the first chakra, you might believe that things are cut-and-dry. Instead of trust being a flowing quality, it stays concrete and categorical. Take for example a two-year-old child, who can change like or dislike of a person depending on an individual experience. If a parent takes away a toy because of bad behavior, the small child might shout out, "I hate you, Daddy!" In that moment, the child feels hate because of a single experience that was displeasing to her. First chakra people behave in a similar way. They tend to be more rigid when it comes to deeper concepts like trust.

But as you move up the chakras, you will notice that things get a little fuzzier, without well-defined boundaries, when it comes to emotional matters. For now, allow yourself to be open to taking steps to trust and see where it takes you.

SECURITY

Tied into trust, feelings of security or lack thereof can be a problem in first chakra balancing. When you experience life through the first chakra alone, you might think you have to do it all alone. You might fall under the illusion that the world is a scary place and you have to fend for yourself or else you will die. (That is, by the way, the essence of survival of the fittest.) Until you can begin thinking otherwise, try living in the present moment. Present-moment awareness is not even a spiritual practice at this point. It simply means looking around you and looking at yourself. Are you living? Are you breathing? Do you have clothes on? Did you have a meal recently? Do you have a roof over your head? Are you okay right now? If so, you are secure.

If you're in a precarious situation, such as being homeless or in an abusive household, go back to the Serenity Prayer. Is there something you can change about your situation? Is there someone you can reach out to?

As you move up through the chakras you will learn that security is elusive. If you seek security for security's sake, you'll never achieve it. The universe is constantly shifting and changing. Wanting security at all costs is essentially the same as wanting to hold on to the universe and hoping it won't change. If you think about it, that's completely absurd. Do what you need to do. Get a job, pay your bills, do good works, give to charity, serve others and the greater good, and that's it. You can't control the rest.

I know a man who was very successful at his job and had

a great salary. All throughout his years at his job he worried constantly that he would be laid off and that his great salary would be taken away. Instead of enjoying his job day to day, being grateful, happy, and joyful, he ruined his everyday life by worrying he would lose it. And do you know what happened? He got laid off. Then he found another great job with a great salary, worried all the time, and got laid off from that job too. Sometimes the act of worrying about security will take away that security.

Deep-seated emotions aren't easy to balance. Without a doubt, it took years to develop these ways of thinking and reacting, and it can take years to change to new ways of thinking. Be patient with yourself as you practice overcoming these first chakra limitations. Take it one step at a time and one day at a time.

 Healing the Spiritual Body

Meditation is a great way to reduce the fight-or-flight response. It teaches you to take a step back from reaction mode. Meditation reduces stress hormones, normalizes blood pressure, reduces heart rate, and improves immune function. When you look at the effects of meditation, you see the complete opposite of the effects of the fight-or-flight response.

Below is a first chakra meditation. You can have someone read it to you while you have your eyes closed; record yourself reading it out loud, and then listen with your eyes closed; or purchase a copy of the audio version of this book and listen to the guided meditations whenever you need them.

MULADHARA GUIDED MEDITATION

Sit comfortably and close your eyes. Make sure your sitting bones are firmly pressed to the floor. To accomplish this, take the fleshy parts of your bottom and bring them out to the sides a little. Inhale deeply through your nose from your lower belly. As you exhale, press the energy downward toward your first chakra as you bring your belly button inward to your spine. Repeat this full, deep breath five times.

Now place your awareness on the root chakra, at the base of your spine. Imagine a swirling, whirling wheel that is deep red in color, spinning around like a planet spinning on its axis. Imagine this powerful energy flowing through you and circulating throughout your perineum, your coccyx, the base of your spine, and your first three vertebrae.

As you breathe deeply, begin to visualize your bottom planting roots deep into the soil. Imagine these roots getting enriched by the fertile earth. You are becoming one with the earth and its magnificent wealth. All the resources you need are here. They are present in the here and now, and they are not far away from you.

In exchange for you trusting the earth in all its wisdom, the earth returns to you the energy you need in the form of vibrations. Feel these vibrations pulsating through your lower body. Welcome them as they bring healing energy to your feet, knees, legs, sciatic nerves, pelvis, and lower back.

Now that your root chakra is awakened, you begin to feel ease and trust that the earth will provide for you in due time. You have planted your roots, like planting seeds in fertile soil, and all you need to do is wait for the seeds to grow into beautiful blossoms. Your worry melts away with each breath. You are grounded. You are safe. You are secure. All your basic needs are met.

Notice how connected you feel to the earth. Notice how your root chakra feels awake and alive. You can enhance the vibrations by chanting the mantra sound *LAM* three times.

ENERGY-BODY HEALING WITH GEMS AND COLORS

To remind yourself to stay grounded, wear the color red, either in your clothing or accessories such as a red bracelet or ribbon. You can also procure red mala beads to wear or hold during your meditation.

Crystals and gems are useful in chakra healing since they carry the earth's energy. First chakra crystals include garnet, red jasper, black tourmaline, and bloodstone.

First Chakra Mindfulness Ideas to Ponder

1. I accept my body as it is. I am grateful for my journey here on earth, and I will immerse myself completely in it. Even though my body appears to be solid, I know it's a constant flow of energy and information. As such, I know my body can always change for the better.
2. I feel connected to the earth and draw energy from it, knowing that Mother Earth provides for me in all her lavish abundance that surrounds me at all times.

3. Today I will connect with nature. I will enhance my sense of smell by taking in the fragrances of flowers, plants, trees, or fresh-cut grass. I will watch animals play, or I will sit down and play with my pets. I will sit on the earth and meditate.

2 THE SACRAL CHAKRA
Svadhisthana

ELEMENT: Water (Jala)
COLOR: Orange
MANTRA SOUND: *VAM*

The word *Svadhisthana* means "sweetness," which is a great way to describe this chakra of attraction. Svadhisthana is the chakra of creativity and sexuality. It is also referred to as the "sacral chakra." It's the second chakra of matter and the point of awakening from the self in survival to the self reaching out toward others. The second chakra is the focal point of pleasure, desire, sexuality, and procreation. While the anatomical region certainly indicates that this chakra is largely focused on sexual matters, matters of creativity are of equal importance. A person who can harness the sexual energy of the second chakra can accomplish great things.

The element of the Svadhisthana chakra is water, or *jala* in Sanskrit. Water is cohesive in nature. It binds, brings together, creates love and devotion, and connects us to one another. Think of the sexual fluids that bind together a woman and man in sexual harmony; these fluids come together to create life. While the first chakra is bound by the earth element, the second chakra has the flowing nature of water.

The anatomical region of the second chakra is the sacral plexus, from the top of the pubic bone up to the navel. It includes the lower abdomen, the genitals, and the womb. The second chakra is also responsible for the bladder and kidneys.

The sense we associate with Svadhisthana is taste, especially the sweet taste. The sense organ is the tongue.

The Ayurvedic dosha corresponding to the second chakra is Kapha, which is composed of water and earth. Svadhisthana is ruled by the guna tamas.

The color we attribute to the sacral chakra is orange. The mantra, or bija (seed) sound, we vocalize for the second chakra is *VAM*.

Second Chakra Ailments

Illnesses and disorders of the second chakra include sexual and reproductive dysfunction such as repeated miscarriages, abortions, frigidity, erectile dysfunction, and premature ejaculation. Second chakra imbalance can also cause uterine, bladder, and kidney problems as well as lower-back stiffness and addictions. Emotional afflictions include eating disorders, low self-esteem, envy, and jealousy.

Second Chakra Energy

Svadhisthana energy comes from the dynamic of its water element and lunar energy. Water plays a big part on our planet and in our bodies. Almost three-fourths of the earth is covered in water and about two-thirds of the human body is made up of water. The moon has a major influence on the tides, our moods, women's menstrual cycles, and even the birth of babies. This dynamic dance between the water element and the moon mirrors the dualistic awakening that happens in the Svadhisthana chakra.

The first chakra energy of survival and its earthly limitations evolves to the second chakra energy of water and the search for connection. The awakened sexual energy leads to desire for earthly pleasures. It's no longer about needing and accumulating things; it's about desire. Food is no longer just a necessity for living; eating becomes a tantalizing sensual experience.

The concept of polarity plays out in the chakras as it does in life. The first chakra carries yang, or masculine energy, and the second chakra carries yin, or feminine energy. Then in the third chakra the energy shifts back to masculine, and so on.

The celestial body of the second chakra is the moon. The energy of the moon is feminine, passive, and changing. Water is the element that gives way to life. The womb of creation, literally and metaphorically, is rooted in the second chakra energy.

Out of the second chakra come music, art, poetry, and dance. Imagination develops in this chakra, as does the deep desire for marriage and family.

Imagine the ebb and flow of the oceans. No longer are we bound to a seemingly solid state where we must find our place. Now we're moved to taste what the earth has to offer. Think of baby sea turtles emerging from their cozy nests in the sand and making their way to the ocean to begin life.

Discovering the second chakra's delights is an exciting awakening. For the first time we experience true duality, in the romantic sense, and we learn the meaning of cause and effect. In the stage of development that corresponds to the second chakra, a baby learns how to playfully manipulate others to get what he wants. When he flirts with his caregivers by performing, laughing, giggling, or repeating some funny antic, he gets hugs, kisses, and much love. We start to learn the effect we have on other people and how to woo them to our side.

The moon energy of the second chakra is a passive but attractive energy. It includes deep emotions, inner strength, nurturing, and nourishing. The mermaid is an archetypal energy of the Svadhisthana chakra. In mythology, mermaids are known for their alluring beauty and melodious voices. Depictions of mermaids show them beautifying themselves by combing their hair and adorning themselves with jewels. They are sexually tantalizing, seductive, and charming as they attract sailors with their luscious song. However, they also have an independent and rebellious side to them, and they only appear by the light of the moon.

Our Societal Relationship with the Second Chakra

In the West, or more particularly in the United States, the predominant lifestyle shows an overindulgence of second chakra pleasures. Everything Americans do is big. We eat large amounts of food, especially in restaurants because they have to give you enough bang for your buck. We are the largest consumers of prescription pills, painkilling medications in particular — we consume 80 percent of the world's supply of opioids. We spend more than $90 billion per year on alcohol consumption. And Americans have on average around $16,601 in credit card debt. We are enthralled with stars and sex symbols, and we attempt to live out pleasures vicariously through them by way of reality TV shows. We are a society of overindulgence.

The concept of delayed gratification holds little ground here. We want things the way we want them, and we want them quickly. The constant search for pleasure and the avoidance of pain, without regard for the consequences, is a second chakra imbalance.

Like the small wooden boy in Disney's *Pinocchio* who is led to Pleasure Island and indulges in many forbidden pleasures but then barely escapes with his life, we too have begun to see consequences of choosing such a lifestyle. Chronic lifestyle diseases such as diabetes, obesity, heart disease, hypertension, stroke, cancer, and alcohol and drug addictions afflict 133 million US adults, or roughly half the adult population. We're getting fatter, sicker, and more addicted by the day.

Pleasure in itself isn't a bad thing. We need to seek out pleasure and avoid pain for our bodies to know that all is well. However, it's the excess that is harmful. It's the inability to overcome the persistent urge to indulge rather than direct this creative energy toward a higher purpose.

Women Working the Second Chakra

Women are readily hardwired for the strengths of second chakra energy. The womb of creation is within them, and they possess the same creative power as the Creator of the universe. This blessed gift gives them the ability to nurture, to be highly sensitive, and to have a heightened sense of intuition. Women are also naturally blessed with the passive inner strength of the second chakra. This strength imbues women with the power of attraction. In mythology, many goddesses are portrayed as passively awaiting good things while adorning themselves with jewels or brushing their thick, luxurious hair. The idea in this portrayal is that the goddess doesn't have to do anything but relax, and like a magnet, she attracts good things to her.

In modern society, women are pulled to live more in yang energy, which is masculine, forward moving, and competitive.

As they compete in the workplace with their male counterparts, they must take on more masculine roles. But in order to remain balanced, all people, women as well as men, must embrace both energies, yin and yang, and problems can result when women move too far into yang energy. Some women feel that they must deny their femininity in certain situations at work or at home, and this can create imbalances. For example, at work a woman might feel compelled to dress more like a man to avoid potential sexual harassment or to fit in a mostly male workplace.

Typically, women who naturally have more yin energy find it easier to swing the pendulum back: they're able to embrace their femininity while performing more masculine activities, and they don't have a difficult time remaining balanced. On the other hand, women who naturally feel more comfortable in a masculine role might not strive to temper their yang energy with their inherent yin.

Health problems can result when women lose this balance. Some women who overidentify with yang energy develop depression, lupus, cancer, high blood pressure, and other diseases. Many others have a hard time getting pregnant. Fertility and procreation are natural when the second chakra is balanced. In fact, they're a normal and healthy part of the process of life. But today, because of the demands of higher education and work, many women wait until after age thirty-five to try to get pregnant. Waiting this long decreases a woman's chance of getting pregnant in the first place. Then, when she finally does get pregnant, she must face the fear of not being on par with her male co-workers because of the physical vulnerability of being pregnant and having a child. So instead of embracing pregnancy as a natural time to enjoy being a woman and to embody goddess energy, she can suppress these feelings in order to fit in.

Excessive yang energy also spills into relationships and family life. Many women are single mothers and must play the role of breadwinner, disciplinarian, homemaker, parent, and head of household. Women who are used to having power and respect in the workplace then take that same yang energy and apply it to parenting and marriage.

The problem is, women aren't physically built to sustain the demands of taking on every single task of both a man and woman, such as working full-time, taking care of a household, creating babies, raising children, being a great wife, balancing the budget, lifting weights five days a week, and volunteering. Wow! It was exhausting just writing all of that. Yet many women are doing all this. In the not-too-distant past, women didn't even handle the traditional household roles alone. They had support networks. Extended family members shared tasks, and the burden was spread across many instead of piled up on one.

Women today feel ashamed that they can't do it all, but they were never meant to. They shouldn't consider it a weakness to need help or to want to embrace their femininity. Women should be proud of their ability to create, to acknowledge their emotions, to be nurturing and sensitive. These are all great qualities. Women shouldn't be afraid to ask for help or admit that they're not Hercules. (You shouldn't be able to carry six grocery bags in one haul.)

I discovered my swelling yang energy when I was learning to dance salsa. I had recently come out of a harsh breakup, and I made the decision to learn how to salsa dance. Partner dancing is very much a second chakra activity. It's flowing, dynamic, and sensual and has a sense of give-and-take. While I fully embrace my feminine side, I am a high-powered woman. I am a single mom. I run my own business, my household, and my life. I'm used to being in control. But whoa, did I learn the hard way that that doesn't work on the dance floor! I took on dance lessons like I take on life. I said to myself, *I'm going to work hard and learn this right. I'm going to be a great dancer, learn the steps, and perfect this.* I was so goal oriented and yang in my thinking, you'd think I was a CEO launching a startup.

Salsa dancing is difficult to learn, but it's not a left-brained activity. It's an art. It's movement and creativity. Supportive — and, I might add, very patient — dance partners taught me how to embrace my second chakra energy. They did this by gently reminding me, "Relax. Let me lead." The first one hundred or so times I danced salsa, I heard that phrase again and again. The funny thing is, I thought I *was* letting them lead. I learned how to be a woman once again on the dance floor. If I hadn't let my dance partners lead, the dynamics of duality and polarity could have never taken place. You can't have two leaders or two followers on the dance floor — it simply doesn't work. The beauty is in yin and yang meshing together perfectly to create the work of art you see in dance competitions.

Women need to decide what energy they truly want to embrace in their relationships. Sometimes I see women who really want to be feminine and act through yin energy, but they don't let themselves, out of fear of being weak. In reality, though, weakness lies only in not knowing who you are or in sending out conflicting messages to the world that don't reflect what you feel inside.

I see this especially in dating. Because they're overidentified with yang energy, many women have become more assertive in dating and in some cases downright aggressive. Traditionally, thanks to his competitive yang nature, a man would want to pursue the woman, woo her, and win her heart. But today, when women take on the yang role, the energetic transfer can take away the man's drive to go out there and work hard to get what he wants.

As a woman, figuring out how to balance your second chakra involves knowing how you would like to embrace your feminine energy so you can keep it open and flowing at all times. Figure out who you are and how you want this energy to manifest, and stick with it. For example, if you've always wanted to be a stay-at-home mom, but family pressures have caused you to remain in a full-time job, you can work toward the role you want to embrace. You could, for example, explore the options of a home-based business working only part-time. I have a friend who ran a home daycare as soon as her first child was born. It allowed her to have income while being able to stay at home with her children. For your own health, try not to let society's expectations get in the way of knowing what's right for you. When you meditate, focus on your second chakra and especially your female sex organs, and ask yourself if you're fully embracing who you are. If you're not, what's holding you back? Stay true to yourself, and you'll find you can more easily become your own best friend.

Living Life in the Svadhisthana Chakra

A person living in the second chakra is like a child exploring the world for the first time without restraint. Imagine the person is a butterfly flitting from flower to flower, tasting, experiencing, and then flying off to experience some more. The words that describe this person are *imagination, emotion*, and *indulgence*.

When it comes to dealing with emotional second chakra people, you'd better watch out. While first chakra people tend to get angry and violent when they're upset, second chakra people throw temper tantrums to get what they want. They sulk, cry, and use emotional blackmail to get their way. You may feel you're on an emotional roller coaster in their presence.

Balanced second chakra people are carefree and imaginative. They like to play out the dramatic role of heroine or dream of being famous actors. They may not have the wherewithal to buckle down and set goals to achieve their dreams, but they talk a good game on how they will be rich and famous. They love art, poetry, and romance.

Like kids in a candy shop, second chakra people tend to overindulge. They overeat, usually eating too many sweets, and indulge in alcohol or drugs. The overindulgence may very well come in other forms such as shopping, gambling, or hoarding. Addictions are typically a problem for people living completely in second chakra energy.

Recognizing Second Chakra Imbalances

When your second chakra is out of balance, it can cause you to be reactive, to get bogged down in deep, dark emotions, and to forget your higher purpose. You can get caught up in emotional battles with yourself or others, which keeps you operating from a low level.

You limit yourself and your Svadhisthana power when you engage in negative self-talk because your emotions tell you, for example, "You screwed up again. You just gained ten pounds"; or when you down an entire bottle of wine because you feel your husband will never understand you; or when you get back at a lover by having sex with someone else.

Also, having shameful feelings about your own sexuality will create blockages and hinder your creativity. Blocking the flow of energy can be as harmful as overindulging in the energy without boundaries.

Accepting Second Chakra Gifts

The gifts you receive from your sacral chakra are perhaps some of the most powerful and transformative gifts of all.

Sex Transmutation

According to Napoleon Hill, author of the world-famous book *Think and Grow Rich*, sexual energy is the most potent energy we possess as humans. He explains that it's the most powerful, motivating, and moving energy if we transmute it wisely — in other words, channel it into other creative pursuits and bring new ideas into being to make the world a better place. And, he continues, if we combine sexual energy with the energy of love (fourth chakra), we can attain anything we put our minds to. He calls this power sex transmutation.

You can channel your sexual energy into any creative activity, whether it's baking a delicious dessert, making a costume, choreographing a dance, or inventing a new electronic device. Entrepreneurs, writers, and scientists are examples of those who know how to successfully use sexual energy by converting it into creative power.

Sexual Intimacy

Using sexual energy for sexual intimacy and pleasure is discussed in the Yoga Sutras of Patanjali. The first yoga sutra presents the yamas, moral precepts for those who wish to live a yogic and disciplined lifestyle. The fourth yama is *bramacharya*. Bramacharya can be interpreted as sexual restraint. The original concept was to refrain from sexual activity to preserve the sexual fluids, known as *shukra* in Sanskrit, to gain greater illumination. In a way, it mirrors the philosophical thought of sex transmutation. Bramacharya was intended to mean that sexual desire is not to be used for selfish and self-serving means. A person who has several sexual partners or goes from one partner to another isn't exercising sexual restraint. The practice of bramacharya means using your sexual energy for sexual pleasure in a committed and intimate partnership, where your concern is to give to your beloved.

Healing Svadhisthana

DAILY AFFIRMATION
I have the right to feel what I feel.
I allow myself to follow my dreams. I deserve pleasure
and goodness in my life. I go with the flow.

 ### Healing the Physical Body

Since so much of the second chakra involves the emotional body, healing your emotions is an integral part of healing Svadhisthana. As we explore second chakra physical healing, I'd like you to think about such things as accepting your gender, your sex organs, the beauty of your physical body, and your sense of taste. While gender and sex aren't the same thing, the polarity of second chakra energy, which includes opposites, indicates gender identity. For example, some women are ashamed of being female and therefore hide their bodies behind unflattering clothes or they hunch their shoulders as they walk or stand. Some men, who may have been beaten down by overbearing mothers, are afraid to show their strength and masculinity.

ENHANCING YOUR SENSE OF TASTE

Your sense of taste is linked to the water element, the Ayurvedic Kapha dosha, and the second chakra. Our sense of taste can become polluted by eating the wrong foods, such as deep-fried, processed, and artificial foods, and by drinking alcohol. Tasting your food is part of the sensual experience of being alive. You can enliven and enhance your sense of taste by swishing with organic food-grade raw sesame oil.

In the first chakra healing section, I suggested eating in silence. You can take this one step further by truly tasting what you're eating and paying close attention to the flavors you enjoy. A good way to wean yourself off junk food is to sit in silence and feel the sensory experience of the unhealthy food. Years ago, I used to eat fast food from time to time. When I noticed the coating of grease stuck to my tongue and teeth or the sugar coating left in my mouth after drinking sugary beverages, I immediately noted that I hated the taste. Then it was easy to let go of those things.

EMBODYING WATER

Second chakra healing practices that involve water or water-like movements can be soothing. Some people are drawn to bodies of water for activities like swimming, surfing, or sailing. Others prefer dancing, tai chi, or qigong. Yoga, especially a slow flow, is great for continual second chakra healing. You will know intuitively which water-like movement practices resonate with you. Choose movements that open your hips, stimulate your internal organs, and strengthen your lower back.

Focusing on Proper Breathing

Most people don't know how to mindfully breathe. Women are taught to suck in their tummies or wear pants that are too tight. Men might tighten their belts to try to look thinner. As a result, many wind up chest-breathing, which creates shallow and panicky breath. As you breathe naturally, your belly should inflate and deflate. This is known as belly-breathing or diaphragmatic breathing, and it involves inhaling from the lower abdomen around the area of the second chakra. You will feel your lower belly puffing out as you inhale properly. To get a full healing breath, refrain from tightening your stomach muscles. Let it all go. Visualize the air circulating freely, in a swirling wheel, throughout your abdomen. As you exhale, you will feel your tummy moving inward, toward your spine. When you shift your breathing in this way, into the area between your pubic bone and belly button, immediately you will feel calmer and more relaxed.

Honoring Your Menstrual Cycle

While this section is dedicated to women, men reading this book can use this knowledge to help and support the women in their lives. We live in a society that is constantly on the go. In the modern world, it's not acceptable to take sick days, slow down, or show lack of drive toward accomplishment. This philosophy goes against the grain of creativity. Creative thought and creative endeavors are best sought out in silence and stillness. Creative energy needs space to move through its channels. When you fill your schedule with too much to do and move full speed ahead, there is no room for space or pause. Women have been blessed with a natural cycle to slow them down at least once a month: their menstrual cycles. Their natural bodily rhythms call for this space in grounding and quietness. A woman's body asks for rest, relaxation, and introspection during the time of menses. If she honors those needs, she will be reinvigorated as a new cycle begins. As a result the second chakra will stay open and aligned. Not only will she experience increased fertility and flow in her life, she will also benefit from increased creativity in the way of abundance and manifestation of desires.

FOODS TO ENHANCE REPRODUCTIVE TISSUE

Ayurvedic remedies to help with fertility and to heal reproductive tissue (*shukra dhatu*) include adding asparagus, broccoli, organic milk, organic fresh dates, organic fresh ripe mangoes, and organic rice pudding to your diet. To reduce toxins before trying to conceive, detox the first and second chakras by taking gentle herbs such as senna or the Ayurvedic formula *triphala*. Spices such as cumin, black cumin, and turmeric are also good for reproductive tissue. These foods and spices will help heal reproductive tissue in both men and women.

YOGA ASANAS AND PRANAYAMA EXERCISES TO HEAL THE SECOND CHAKRA

Yin yoga is a great style of yoga to help balance the second chakra. The idea behind yin yoga is to keep the body cool by doing slow movements and holding the poses for three to five minutes each. During a yin class, you're assisted with yoga props such as blocks, blankets, bolsters, and straps. A set of yin yoga poses assists in opening your hips and working your connective tissue. The poses below are yin poses, except the last one, dhanurasana. I've included dhanurasana, a yang pose, because it helps bring vibrant energy to the second chakra.

To view a video demo of these exercises, go to
www.youtube.com/c/MichelleFondinAuthor.
Click on the Playlists tab, and select
Chakra Healing Asanas & Pranayamas.
Scroll down the list until you find the one you're looking for.

Left-Nostril Breathing — *Ida Nadi Pranayama*: Sit tall and place your left hand on your lap. Place the index and middle finger of your right hand on your right nostril to close it. Slowly inhale and exhale through your left nostril only. Do this breathing technique for a minute or two.

Cow and Cat Poses: On all fours, spread out your fingers on the floor and flex your toes. As you inhale, lift your tailbone up toward the sky, raise your head and look up, and lower your belly toward the floor. As you exhale, draw your belly button in toward your spine and your chin down toward your chest, lower your tailbone, and raise your spine into a curve, like an angry Halloween cat. Do eight sets of cow and cat.

Pigeon Pose — *Eka Pada Rajakapotasana*: From your all-fours position, slide your right knee forward, and set it down in front of your left knee. Bring your right heel forward, away from your pelvis as much as possible. Extend your left leg all the way behind you, and set your left foot on the floor as you bring your hips close to the floor. Come down to your elbows and rest your forehead down. If your hips are tight, you can place a bolster or pillow underneath your right hip. Hold for three minutes, then switch to the other side.

Cobra Pose — *Bhujangasana*: Lie flat on your belly. Slide your feet together so your big toes touch. Place your forehead to the floor. With your palms on the floor, bring your fingers slightly behind your shoulders with your elbows bent. Squeeze your bottom, and press your pubic bone toward your mat. Bring your shoulders back and away from your ears. Press down on your hands, and hug your elbows against your torso to lift your head and upper chest off the floor. Be mindful of your feet and make sure they stay on the floor. If you're doing this properly, you should feel this pose in your lower back (area of the second chakra) and triceps. To make the pose a yin pose, as you lift your head and chest, set your elbows down underneath your ribs and place your hands and forearms down on the mat, like a sphinx. Relax your shoulders down, and breathe as you stimulate your lower belly and lower back. Hold for two minutes.

Happy Baby Pose — *Yoga Nidrasana*: Have you ever seen a baby hold his feet and giggle happily on his back? That's the idea of the happy baby pose. On your back, lift your legs up and bend your knees, drawing your knees and feet wide apart. Hold the outer edges of your flexed feet with your hands. It will look like an upside-down squatting posture. If you can't clasp your feet, hold on to your ankles or calves. To stimulate your kidneys, inhale deeply and hold your breath. Still holding your breath, rock side to side six to eight times, then exhale as you come back to the center. Repeat the series two to three times.

Reclining Bound-Angle Pose / Reclining Butterfly Pose — *Supta Baddha Konasana*: Lie on your back. Bring the soles of your feet together as your knees open wide, into a butterfly shape. Allow your hips to relax completely. If the stretch is too intense, you can place yoga blocks underneath your knees. Place your hands on your belly, and focus on your breath. Hold the pose for three to five minutes.

Bow Pose — *Dhanurasana*: Start on your belly with your arms at your sides. Bring your feet up into the air, and reach up to catch them with your hands. You can take hold of your feet or your ankles. Lift your head and chest, and breathe deep into your lower belly. A deep rhythmic breath will create a rocking motion and will stimulate your internal organs. This is also a great pose to do for menstrual cramps. Hold the pose for one to two minutes and repeat two to three times.

 ## Healing the Emotional and Energetic Body

From repressed sexuality to low self-esteem to overindulgence, issues surrounding the emotional body of the second chakra are many. Healing this area will help you overcome many emotional scars and advance in your emotional and spiritual journey.

BUILDING SELF-ESTEEM

Good self-esteem can be a result of nature and nurture. Sometimes children who grow up in the same family have varied levels of self-esteem. Other times, low self-esteem seems to result from abandonment or emotional or physical abuse in childhood. No matter the cause, it can be challenging to build self-esteem back up to normal levels.

The practice of yoga, including a focus on chakra healing, can help raise self-esteem. People with low self-esteem are constantly seeking approval from others. This is known as *object referral*. Object referral says, "I'm valuable because of what I do, who loves me, or what I have." Right or wrong, it's what happens. But in reality, it's impossible to please or impress everyone — one hundred people will have one hundred different opinions of you — and to even try to do so is exhausting. Self-referral, on the other hand, says, "I'm valuable because I'm an integral part of this great big universe. I'm needed and wanted because I'm here. God, Mother Nature, or my Higher Power is in me, and I hold the same creative essence that is contained in them." When you assimilate yoga practices and philosophy, you begin to shift your focus from object referral to self-referral. When this shift happens, you have an aha moment —you finally realize that everything you have been striving for in the way of approval (and, of course, falling short) is an unattainable goal. You're already perfect as you are.

Become your best friend. Before you say something to yourself or think something about yourself, ask if you would say it to your best friend.

Nurturing Yourself

Take care of your body as a good mother would take care of her child. She makes sure the child is eating three to five times per day and getting plenty of nutrients. She ensures the child gets enough rest. She takes her child out for walks daily. She caresses and strokes her child's skin and reassures her child when she's frightened. She makes sure her child has time for play, work, and friends. A good mother takes her child for wellness checkups and gives her vitamins to grow. Take care of yourself in all the same ways.

Nurturing is a second chakra trait. You will enhance your second chakra energy when you nurture yourself.

Healing from Addictions

People who suffer from addiction, in any form, have a second chakra imbalance. Addicts seek pleasure through the object of addiction at all costs. They will charm and deceive others to get that object. Like second chakra energy, there is a sense of reaching out toward others, but the goal isn't for connection and love in the higher sense of the chakra but rather to attain a temporary fix for a transcendent moment in bliss. However, all false attempts to reach transcendence and enlightenment by destructive means create karmic debt and leave the user in a deeper hole of indebtedness each time.

I'm very much attached to the subject of addiction because I have a loved one who suffers from alcoholism. I became so entrenched in the study of alcoholism that I wrote a book about it titled *Help! I Think My Loved One Is an Alcoholic: A Survival Guide for Lovers, Family, and Friends.* I'm a firm believer in 12-step programs for any addiction. Some addictions may be healed through practices such as meditation and yoga, but as one of my friends in recovery told me, the -ism is still there. Addiction doesn't happen overnight, and it's not undone overnight. If you or someone you love suffers from addiction, I highly recommend getting professional help in addition to using chakra-based healing or other holistic and spiritual practices.

EMOTIONAL HEALING

Mind-body connection in health is undeniable. Study after study, including one published in the January 11, 2017, issue of *The Lancet*, shows that emotional health can have as much of an impact on your heart health as tobacco use or obesity. Doing emotional health exercises is just as useful as physical exercise. Those who aren't hardwired with an optimistic emotional outlook may need to practice increasing emotional health daily to strengthen those muscles.

Here are a few things you can try daily:

- Say, chant, or write positive affirmations, and refrain from negative self-talk.

- Write your thoughts down in a journal.
- Have in-person experiences with good friends and not simply online relationships.
- Volunteer your time once a week or once a month.
- Keep a gratitude journal: on a regular basis, write down the things you're grateful for.

 ## Healing the Spiritual Body

Aligning with and accepting your power of creation can help heal your second chakra spiritual energy. Your power to create was freely given to you by your Creator and therefore is good. In healing the second chakra, we work to overcome limiting beliefs about our sexuality and creativity.

Sexuality

Religious interpretation of sexual intimacy has given this natural, human, and God-given act a dirty name. The many words we hear in religious circles around sex include *shameful, dirty, sinful,* and *lustful.* I believe this creates a shadow energy around sexuality and vilifies it. As a result, people sneak around behind closed doors and talk about sexual intimacy in hushed tones. This aura of oppression can cause people to act toward extremes and wreak havoc on relationships.

I personally don't believe that the Creator of the universe, who gave us consciousness and conscious awareness of love and intimacy, intended for it to be this way. To heal your sexual energy, you may need to shift your thinking and behavior toward a healthier pathway.

The Western interpretation of Tantra or Tantric sex, in its purest meaning, gives a clearer picture of a more spiritual experience with sex. We are different from other animals in that we have the capacity to control and modify our emotions, breath, bodily functions, and connection to each other and to spirit. We have the choice to act differently than with the instinctual and hardwired reactions programmed in our brains by our predecessors.

From my understanding in connection with yoga, which means "to yoke," "to unite," or "to join together," the act of sexual intimacy can be spiritual in nature, as a way to honor the body, mind, soul, and spirit of your partner and vice versa. In accordance with *bramacharya*, this union is best explored in a committed, exclusive, and long-term relationship. Instead of pure mechanical performance, so to speak, spiritual sexual intimacy brings more awareness to the physical connection. It involves taking the time to get to know your partner on every level and arriving at the level of vulnerability needed to create union in a yogic sense of the word. The act of lovemaking can be a truly transcendent experience.

In this understanding of transcendent sexuality, you wouldn't want to take lovemaking lightly, but instead come at it from a vantage point not of shame but of purity — a sense of purity that comes from within you, as a true recognition of the gift your sexuality brings, rather than an idea imposed on you from someone or something external. When you assimilate this understanding into your being, you won't want to squander your sexual energy on a subpar or purely physical experience.

Some of the things you might want to explore within yourself as you look toward healing the sexual power of your second chakra are the following:

1. What is my view of my own sexuality?
2. What was I taught about sexuality growing up?

3. Have I ever given away my body to another because of demands put upon me?
4. Have I ever had a sexually intimate experience in which I felt connected to my partner in body, mind, soul, and spirit?
5. Have I ever used sex to get what I want?
6. Has my view of sexual intimacy changed over the years?
7. Have I had physical symptoms in my second chakra as a result of my beliefs about my sexuality? (Examples are lower back pain, uterine problems, erectile dysfunction, and ovarian cysts.)
8. How will I change my view of my own sexuality to help heal my second chakra?

CREATIVITY

As I was growing up, I thought the creative gene had been given only to my sister, who was naturally artistic. I looked at my scribbles and stick-figure drawings and felt destined to a life of desk work and intellectual pursuits.

Yet as I grew up I learned I did have some creativity in my genes. After all, writing is creative. But I also love to bake, cook, and dance. Creating is all about taking raw materials that you know, such as words or food ingredients, and putting them together to create something new. So even if you're an accountant and have discovered a more efficient way to enter numbers, you're a creator.

That being said, awakening the creative energy of the second chakra is about opening yourself to the creative mind of the universe to assist you along the way. Napoleon Hill in *Think and Grow Rich* says, "The great artists, writers, musicians, and poets become great because they acquire the habit of relying upon the 'still small voice' which speaks from within, through the faculty of creative imagination." He explains that this creative imagination, also known as "hunches," is only obtained through four sources: infinite intelligence, one's subconscious mind, the mind of another person, or another person's subconscious mind. He explains that genius is only released through this method and that most people don't access this incredible force during the entire span of their lifetime. I'm reminded of the great Walt Disney, who, despite major failures and setbacks, worked the second chakra in a positive way to create magic for families across the globe.

Taking a break from daily monotony to do something creative can allow your imagination to run wild. Daydreaming, imagining, and mind wandering are wonderful ways to create anything you desire. As speaker and author Tony Robbins says, "Everything in your external world started in your internal world."

Today, take thirty minutes out of your day to do something creative. Turn off all electronic devices, and give your imagination free rein. Become immersed in the creative flow.

SVADHISTHANA GUIDED MEDITATION

Wearing clothing that allows you to breathe fully into your lower belly, sit comfortably with your eyes closed. Take a couple of deep inhalations and deep exhalations, imagining the breath circulating throughout the area of the second chakra.

Visualize a deep orange color moving in a spinning motion, like a disk, cleansing the area above the pubic bone and below the navel. Imagine this spinning disk catching debris, toxins, and any other negative impressions left in the Svadhisthana chakra. Imagine the disk, like a magnet, attracting all negative and clogged energy from your bladder, sex organs, lower back, and pelvis. Once the spinning orange disk has collected all debris from the second chakra, it now pulverizes that negativity and turns it into dust. That dust will be eliminated through your excretory system. Now your second chakra is free from all blockages and negativity.

Next, imagine beautiful, cleansing water such as clear ocean water moving through the second chakra, polishing it and making it like new. Imagine the swishing sound as the salt water flows throughout, bringing harmony back to your creativity chakra.

You are now ready to move into a higher aspect of second chakra energy. You are freed from addictions, lust, cravings, low self-esteem, sexual dysfunction, and infertility. You are now ready and open to create whatever it is that you desire. You are free to create a baby, a new job, a new home, a new relationship, a new company, or a new work of art. Whatever you can imagine, you can achieve. Your creative energy is at one with the creative mind of the universe. In your healing, you draw from this energy, the energy of Source. Creativity flows through you and outward. You are infinite possibilities.

Notice how connected you feel to the water element. Notice how awake and alive your creativity chakra feels. You can enhance the vibrations by chanting the mantra sound *VAM* three times.

ENERGY-BODY HEALING WITH GEMS AND COLORS

You can remind yourself to focus on second chakra healing by wearing the color orange or surrounding yourself with orange objects throughout the day.

The gemstones for this chakra are amber, orange calcite, citrine, and orange aventurine.

Second Chakra Mindfulness Ideas to Ponder

1. Affirmation: I am strong and healthy. I am valuable and perfect the way I am. I am a creative force like the One who created me.

2. I will spend part of my day near a water source — a flowing fountain, a pond, a river, a stream, or the ocean — or I will immerse myself in water sounds such as falling rain or ocean waves. As I listen to and experience the power of water, I will imagine the fluidity of my own body. Even though it's seemingly solid, it's ever flowing and transforming.

3. I will embrace the power of lunar energy and its cycles of waxing and waning. I know that I too have cycles within my body, and I respect those cycles. I will respect my need for rest and relaxation as well as activity. I will align myself with the earth's cycles of day and night and the changing of the seasons, and in so doing I will move with the creative flow of the universe.

4. I will respect my need to play, dance, sing, paint, bake, and express myself and my body in creative ways. I know that giving in to this carefree side of who I am will create balance in my life.

3 THE SOLAR PLEXUS CHAKRA
Manipura

ELEMENT: Fire (Tejas)
COLOR: Yellow
MANTRA SOUND: *RAM*

The third chakra is called Manipura, and the translation is "lustrous gem" or "the dwelling place of the self." The Manipura chakra is strong and important as it represents the emergence of personality into the outer world. It's the seat of the ego. The element and planet of the third chakra go hand in hand, as the element is fire and the planet is the sun. The physical location of the Manipura chakra is the solar plexus, the area just above the navel. Imagine Manipura as a bright yellow sun shining outward and showing itself to the world. The pancreas, adrenal glands, digestive system, and diaphragm and psoas muscles are all a part of the solar plexus chakra. The sense for Manipura is sight, and the sense organ is the eye.

The third chakra is the last of the chakras of physical matter. The lessons we learn from the first three chakras help us move into higher planes where opportunities for spiritual awakening exist. Many stay stuck in the lessons of the first three chakras, repeating them time and again but not necessarily learning how to reap the benefits of these energies from a higher perspective. Certainly it's easy to slip up from time to time, but if you learn how to transcend the limitations of the chakras of matter, you will be able to change and evolve so that the next time a problem arises you handle it differently. And that is truly what the third chakra represents — transformation.

Manipura is our center of personal power. When this chakra is properly open and aligned, we feel a sense of power in our actions. We feel we can effectively manifest our needs and desires, and make a difference in our lives. When balanced, Manipura's power brings about change and forward movement to achieve goals. Imbalanced, it generates self-serving or ineffective actions.

The Ayurvedic dosha for the third chakra is Pitta (fire and water), and the guna is rajas.

The color we attribute to the solar plexus chakra is yellow like the sun. The mantra, or bija (seed) sound, we vocalize for the third chakra is *RAM*.

Third Chakra Ailments

Diseases of the third chakra may include diabetes or other diseases of the pancreas, ulcers, hypoglycemia, digestive disturbances such as irritable bowel syndrome, digestive tract dysfunctions, and diseases of the liver and kidneys. Mental ailments include a severe chemical form of depression with suicidal tendencies.

Third Chakra Energy

The desires for prominence, importance, and success are all part of third chakra energy. A strong Manipura chakra will have you shine brightly to the world. While the second chakra has yin, or female energy, the third chakra has yang, or masculine energy. Linked to the Ayurvedic mind-body type Pitta, which is composed of fire and water, third chakra energy is about the sun's heat, brilliance, and vibrancy.

The sun is bright, shiny, beautiful, and warm. It's also penetrating, constant, and nourishing. The energy of the sun makes people driven, goal oriented, passionate, and brilliant. People embodying the sun's energy will strive hard and never quit. However, the sun can also be hot, overbearing, too bright, scorching, and unrelenting, and people who are too driven by solar energy can display these qualities. They might be quick to anger, hotheaded, overimposing, or critical.

As with all energies, you can use third chakra energy for positive or negative ends, depending on your perspective. Let's suppose you must finish a work project. You need Manipura's inner drive and boundless energy to complete the project. However, if you use it to boss people around, criticize, and point out that your way is better, you may be using it in the negative.

Inner Power

To achieve any task, you need drive, focus, and discipline. Your drive comes from desire and will. Focus allows you to move ahead in your task without distractions. Discipline is the willpower to put together drive and focus to reach your goal.

Personal power reflects healthy development of the third chakra. Take, for example, a child whose sense of self emerges and who begins to express himself as separate from his parents. Loving parents will view his sense of individuality and independence as normal development. They will lovingly guide him while letting him have his own personal preferences and desires, which may or may not match theirs. This child will grow up to have a positive sense of self and will not be afraid to take risks and assert himself. He will be able to effectively stand out from the crowd and trust his own judgment versus blindly following out of fear. On the other hand, parents who aren't psychologically healthy will look at a child's sense of independence as a threat and may squelch his need to differentiate himself. These parents will create unhealthy ties through guilt trips, shame, and codependent behaviors. They will refuse to cut the umbilical cord, so to speak. A child who grows up in this kind of environment will have difficulty asserting his will and knowing what he wants to do in life to celebrate his unique talents. He may be afraid to stand out from the crowd. As an adult, this child may feel disempowered or choose friends and lovers who contribute to this sense of disempowerment by dominating over him. In adulthood, he will need to work through those third chakra issues, formed in early childhood, to take ownership of his inner power.

Willpower

From inner power arises willpower. Carnal and material desires, formulated in the second chakra, are held in check by the third. Willpower says, "I will not have that second piece of cake" or "I need to stay faithful to my spouse despite the fact that this attractive person is coming on to me." Willpower helps create the focus needed to manifest desires with one-pointed attention. For me it says, "I will spend two hours daily writing this book regardless of all the distractions in my life." Your inner fire comes forth to forge the pathway toward your destiny. Strong willpower helps you delay gratification. This shows a personal evolution from second chakra energy and its tendency toward impulsiveness and immediate gratification. People who harness the willpower energy of the third chakra can accomplish great things personally and to help others. Inner power and will-power combined give us our sense of positive self-worth. They tell us what we want and how to get it.

Radiant You

You can use third chakra energy to stand out from the crowd like a beacon. When you're using it in the positive, you rise above as a shining example for your friends, family, and peers. Often through achievements in school, work, or athletic com-petition, those working the positive Manipura energy will be inspirations for those looking to attain the same goals. How-ever, if your drive is to seek approval for the sake of being put up on a pedestal, you will constantly fall short and seek more until you fall completely, often from a state of exhaustion. Even in great accomplishments there must be a higher purpose to balance out the temporary high of rising to the top.

We have all heard stories of film or sports celebrities who rise to the top and have everything, only to fall from grace, lose all their money, or become entrapped in the clutches of ad-diction. This also happens in everyday life to ordinary people who succeed in getting the top salary, opulent house, luxury car, or ideal family, only to realize that they're fundamentally unhappy. Without a higher sense of purpose, we all see our bright lights go out. At this point, the link to the higher chakras becomes indispensable.

Our Societal Relationship with the Third Chakra

If we were to place the United States, as a country, into a chakra energy, the third one would be it. We are a country of overachievers, constantly on the go. We demand that stores be open 24/7, and we want everything bigger, better, faster, and stronger. We also tend to be a society of individuals climbing some invisible ladder. Sometimes, particularly in corporate America, we strive to outshine one another and even "scorch" the competition. As you look at the history of the United States, it makes sense that we embody third chakra energy. We were a fiery people who stood up against the status quo. Our ancestors rebelled against oppressive governments and monarchies and religious persecution. Many immigrants today were strong enough to escape the strongholds of political corruption or chaos and sought freedom in a better land. As a society, we are driven.

The United States was built on the gifts, talents, and inner drive of all who came here to create a better life. Yet this burning desire didn't come without cost. The decimation of the American Indian population, their culture, and their land has created a karmic debt that needs to be repaid. If you look today at the greed that is driving the depletion of the earth's natural resources, and the rewards given for more competition and accumulation of material items, you can see how the fire element's transformative effects can consume us.

This drive has taken its toll. American people are among the sickest and most addicted in the world. Unless we rebalance the scales, the United States cannot move forward with positive power to make the world a better place.

Other modern societies are certainly suffering similar consequences of inner fire power gone wild. They too will need to face the fact that shifting toward more balance is the only way to survive.

Men Working the Third Chakra

Mother Nature gave men natural yang and third chakra energy. Traditionally throughout time, men were hunters, gatherers, protectors of family, warriors, and leaders. Women, with natural yin energy, were nurturers, caretakers, homemakers, healers, and creators. Men were admired in tribes and ancient societies as protectors and heroes. This gave their egos the much-needed boost to continue the job of going out into the wilderness, putting their lives in danger, and fighting to protect what was theirs.

Modern society, for the most part, has taken away this role, leaving men lost and confused. I've talked to many young men and even older men who say they can't figure out their role in family life and in romantic partnership. Their inner drive says to be the head of the house, the breadwinner, the protector, and the chivalrous knight. But the women in their lives seem to be domineering, headstrong, and inconsistent in articulating their desires. With two-income households, the gift men traditionally provided through monetary contribution is no longer seen as special. As women become physically stronger through kickboxing, weight training, or other intense workouts, men have lost their role as protector. Artificial insemination has even made men insignificant in parenthood. Indeterminate guidelines have diminished men's roles in society. Like women who have moved into a more masculine role, men have to figure out how to honor their true nature while keeping in mind the expectations of modern life.

Balanced third chakra energy is about honoring who you truly are. Men, as well as women, can't be afraid to express who they are inside. Denial is dangerous. As a forty-six-year-old woman who has raised two boys while living married, unmarried, and dating, I want to encourage my male readers: be proud of your masculinity and what that means to you. People will respect you more when you stand in your personal power. If you want to pay for dates, open doors, and carry groceries, do it. If you want to stay at home with the kids while your spouse goes to work, own it. And if you're happy being the breadwinner and protector, find a partner who honors that. In other words, don't change who you are because society has changed. We need more men who are willing to stand in their truth and be the men they want to be.

Living Life in the Manipura Chakra

People who are stuck in the third chakra may be accused of being ego-centered. A child who passes through this stage is absorbed with "me" and "mine." If you try to take her toy, she will grab it back and say, "Mine!" The child is trying to define herself as separate from her parents and caretakers. Adults with this mind-set believe they're the center of the universe. They're the sun and everyone else revolves around them. For better and for worse, they take everything personally. They shine brightly because they attempt to impress others. However, if you get on their bad side, they will burn you, like the heat of the sun. They begin and end their conversations with the word *I*, as they like to talk about themselves.

Another subgroup that naturally seems to embody third chakra energy is adolescents. They're absorbed with fashion and physical appearance and fascinated with pop icons and TV celebrities. They become self-conscious if they don't have the right clothes, and they can feel judged by peers for not fitting in.

Those who live from this state of consciousness base their happiness on others' reactions and their own popularity. They crave approval from others and go to great lengths to get it. However, if you don't approve of them or give them accolades, they will either fall into depression or become critical of you for not seeing them as great.

Third chakra people may be labeled as workaholics or type A personalities because they always seem to be chasing an unattainable goal. The goal may be status, money, recognition, or fame. Yet when they attain it, dissatisfaction arises because they always seem to want more to quench the thirst for approval and acknowledgment.

Recognizing Third Chakra Imbalances

The ego is a part of us. It represents our sense of self in this world. In many Eastern philosophies and even in Western psychology, the ego is seen as something bad. Ayurveda, however, sees the ego as an integral part of who we are. I subscribe to the Ayurvedic theory, and it's something I've taught in my meditation courses for many years.

Yoga philosophy teaches that we have layers to our existence. We have three macro layers: the physical body, the subtle body, and the causal body. Each of these macro layers is made up of micro layers. The physical body is composed of the environment, the body, and the energy body, which includes the chakras. The subtle body is composed of the mind, the intellect, and the ego. The causal body includes the individual soul, the collective soul, and the universal soul. All these layers are absolutely necessary to make up who we are as people. No one layer is more important than another.

If these somewhat esoteric layers are difficult for you to grasp, think of your life and the roles you play. As a woman, you might play the roles of daughter, sister, mother, or wife.

You might play the role of someone who works, goes shopping, gives advice to a friend, and has hobbies. As a man, you might be a son, father, brother, or husband. You might be someone who programs computers, plays sports, volunteers for a charity, or plays video games. All these roles are integral parts of who you are as a person. While one role might take precedence over another at any given moment in your life, no single role can eclipse all the others.

Many people come to a spiritual practice, such as yoga, with the mind-set of "I must get rid of the ego and be a totally spiritual person." This mind-set tends to create imbalances and must be approached with caution.

The ego is your personality in society. It represents your sense of individuality and uniqueness. Self-esteem and self-worth emanate from your ego. Your sense of personal power and accomplishment come from ego consciousness. If you play any role in relationships with others and in society, you must embrace your ego as your friend. For example, in searching for a job you need to point out why you're a better candidate than others. You need to have the self-awareness and self-confidence to point out your strengths, talents, and experience. When you're dating with the goal of finding a life partner, you need your ego not only to attract a potential mate but also to win him or her over. Do you see how it's nearly impossible to go through life denying your ego?

However, your ego can be problematic when it takes over and you operate *only* from ego consciousness. Sometimes we can get into the mode of only looking out for our own needs, wants, and desires and forgetting that everyone around us is trying to do the same. You can recognize this limitation and try to move beyond it by bringing awareness to your ego. Notice when you are being self-centered or selfish. Become a detective and find out why. If you naturally tend to think of yourself first, override that by finding out what the other person wants first or making the decision to take turns. Or perhaps you're acting out of ego consciousness because you used to deny your needs and desires and now you're fed up. Whatever the reason, honor your ego's messages and take action to bring balance to the situation.

Accepting Third Chakra Gifts

Become a shining example of who you are. While you can use your third chakra gifts to move yourself ahead in life, you can also use them to help make others' lives better. You can use your inner drive to create a movement or to protest injustice, to contribute to a charity or cause, or to start your own business. Inner power is a gift. Your inner power will allow you to stand up for your beliefs, defend those who need it, and rise up against those who might harm you.

Gifts of the Manipura chakra will allow you to set boundaries and be assertive. These are all positive aspects that delineate you from me and that will, in the long run, create more positive and fulfilling relationships in every aspect of your life.

Healing Manipura

DAILY AFFIRMATION
I stand firm in my personal power
as a shining example for others.
I am certain of my wants, needs, and desires.

Healing the Physical Body

During our time in our mother's womb, we were nourished through the umbilical cord. We received all our sustenance through this cord. This constant nourishment left us lacking for nothing, and when it got cut, our journey to separateness in our physical existence began. The symbolic moment of the cord cutting is intimately linked to third chakra development. In the course of those nine months, we were given everything we needed to survive and thrive on this journey of life on earth. Assuming we have developed normally both physically and mentally, we have a body and mind that work. In our separateness, we can then figure out our mission for the next hundred years or so.

The trust built in the first chakra and the desires of the second chakra lead us to the drive and power of the third. These three forces come together to propel us to work, create the life we desire, and begin to fulfill our life purpose.

Interestingly, we continue to receive nourishment from the same area of the body as before the umbilical cord was cut. The third chakra is the seat of digestion. Ayurveda describes *agni*, or the digestive force, as the ultimate way to determine a person's health. *Agni* means "fire," and healthy agni allows us to assimilate the nutrients we consume into vital energy to move through life. Healthy agni also helps us digest emotions and experiences. The health of your digestive fire will determine how you go through each day. In the physical body, you strengthen your solar plexus chakra through proper nutrition and exercises to enhance your inner fire.

PROPER DIGESTION AND ASSIMILATION OF NUTRIENTS

Ayurveda teaches much about creating healthy agni. When your agni is strong, you create healing chemicals called *ojas*.

Weak agni produces toxins called *ama*. Eating clean and whole foods helps you create a healthy digestive system. Refrain from eating processed, artificial, and chemically produced food. As much as you're able, eat organic food. Balance your diet by eating fruits and vegetables that have naturally vibrant colors, such as the deep red and purple pigments of eggplant, red onions, and tomatoes; the dark greens of kale, collard greens, and spinach; or the deep orange hues of pumpkin, butternut squash, oranges, and carrots.

For proper digestion, minimize raw foods, and lightly cook or sauté vegetables. During meals avoid drinking beverages other than room-temperature water, and make sure you're eating in a calm environment. Ayurveda also suggests eating freshly cooked food at every meal versus eating leftovers and reheated food.

Yoga Asanas and Pranayama Exercises to Heal the Third Chakra

It's relatively easy to balance the third chakra through movement and breathing. You can enhance your digestion and bring health to the Manipura chakra simply by walking for ten minutes after each meal.

> To view a video demo of these exercises, go to
> **www.youtube.com/c/MichelleFondinAuthor**.
> Click on the Playlists tab, and select
> **Chakra Healing Asanas & Pranayamas**.
> Scroll down the list until you find the one you're looking for.

Bellows Breath — *Bhastrika*: Translated as "bellows breath," *bhastrika* is a way to create heat in the body. You can also use this breathing technique if you're trying to lose weight. To practice bhastrika, sit on the floor cross-legged or in a chair with your feet flat on the floor, spine tall, and shoulders relaxed. You will be breathing through your nose with your lips closed. Place your awareness on the area around your belly button and diaphragm. To begin, inhale passively through your nose, and exhale forcefully while contracting your belly in toward your spine. Then inhale forcefully as you puff out your belly. Continue to forcefully exhale and inhale in one-second increments. You can even say quietly to yourself *one-two-one-two-one-two*. After about ten seconds, take a break and take in a deep inhalation and exhalation. Then begin a second set of bhastrika. Practice bhastrika for one to two minutes. When you're finished, it may feel as if you have done many sets of abdominal exercises.

Boat Pose — *Navasana*: Sit tall with your knees bent and feet flat on the floor. If you're working on a hard surface, sit on a folded blanket. Find a focal point ahead, and fix your gaze at about eye level. With your arms beside you, hold on to the backs of your thighs. When you feel centered, lift your feet off the ground. Straighten your legs as much as you're able — it's okay to keep your knees slightly bent if necessary. When you feel ready, let go of your thighs and extend your arms in front of you. Your torso and legs will be in a *V* shape. Even though you will be leaning backward, lengthen through your back. Hold the pose as long as you can. To release from navasana, hold on to your legs once again and lower your feet toward the floor.

Plank Pose: Begin on all fours with your hands right below your shoulders and your knees about hip-width apart. Extend your right leg straight back, and place the ball of your foot down. Then extend your left leg and place that foot down so that both legs are straight. Keep your hips level to the floor; try not to overcompensate by raising your hips too high or sinking your hips too low. When you're doing plank properly, you will feel the intense fire in your belly. Breathe deeply. If you can only hold it for a second or two in the beginning, lower one knee to the floor at a time. Then repeat the exercise three to four times.

Sun Salutations — *Surya Namaskar*: As the name suggests, Sun Salutations give a salute to the sun. This classical series of twelve yoga poses lengthens and strengthens every major muscle group in the body. This flow is done repetitively to enhance flexibility, strength, and cardiovascular health. You can find many variations of the Sun Salutations, and there is no one correct way of doing them.

 Healing the Emotional and Energetic Body

Standing in personal power is more difficult for some than for others. Difficulties may stem from upbringing or personality. For example, growing up with abusive, dysfunctional, or overly authoritarian parents may have given you fears about standing in your personal power. Or maybe you never learned to stand up for yourself and your beliefs. Or maybe you're a naturally shy person and you've never been good at asserting yourself. But no matter the cause, you can get better at claiming your personal power.

BOUNDARIES

Boundary setting is an important part of manifesting your third chakra energy. When you set respectful boundaries, you are saying to others, "I know who I am, and I am proud. I feel confident, and I can respectfully say no when it's appropriate." People with poor boundaries or no boundaries may come off as aggressive, angry, and critical because they aren't able to effectively draw the line between what's theirs and what's not. As a result, they tend to take on other people's problems, issues, and responsibilities, and then they blow up when they've had enough.

Poor boundaries come from low self-esteem. Those who don't effectively set boundaries are afraid of not being liked. Many of their actions don't come from a place of power but from a place of feeling powerless.

People pleasing is one manifestation of weak boundaries. It involves hiding your true wants, needs, and desires or suppressing them so that others can get what they want and/or so that they like you. While it may seem kindhearted, people pleasing is dishonest and even manipulative. If you're a people pleaser, you might wonder why people don't respect you. It's because everyone has needs, and others intuitively know this. People who buy into your people pleasing are generally operating from their egos. They will get what they want from you when they want it, and they know it. But those people need boundaries too. Boundaries show that you have enough respect for yourself not to be a doormat.

Second, people pleasing and poor boundary setting will never give you your personal power. Giving in for the sake of being nice can leave you with frustration and resentment. You can learn to set boundaries by being assertive in response to others' requests rather than responding with negativity. For example, if a good friend has asked you, yet again, to borrow money to pay for dinner and has never paid you back, you could set a boundary by saying, "I will do it this time. But I want to let you know that this is the last time I lend you money." In this case, although it would be easy for you to get angry at your friend or criticize her, by stating what you are willing to do or not willing to do and sticking to it, you will feel empowered without causing negative feelings.

ASSERTIVENESS

Growing up with a domineering mother, I wasn't always assertive. My great moments of embarrassment as a child came when she frequently returned items at stores when she had overspent. She would literally badger the salesperson with every story in the book and even resort to tears to get her way. When I would ask her why she behaved that way, because it was so embarrassing to me, she responded that she was simply being assertive. I thought, *If that's assertive, I will never be assertive in my life.* After growing up and eventually realizing that what she did wasn't assertiveness but manipulation, I slowly learned how to not be a doormat.

To develop and heal your sense of personal power, you can learn how to be assertive without being manipulative. One simple way to practice assertiveness is by saying no. If someone asks you to do something that you don't want to do, you can respond by saying no. You don't even have to qualify that no. Those of us who have poor boundaries have a tough time saying the word *no* as a complete sentence and without explanation. People who are strong in their personal power have no issues with saying no. Other variations of *no* might include "I'm sorry, I can't," "I'm busy that day," or "Not right now."

Successful boundary setters also stick to their decisions and refrain from flip-flopping. If you say no but then allow the person in front of you to persuade you to change your mind, you're not sticking to your boundaries.

Another frequent problem with lack of assertiveness is denying your needs. Have you ever had a friend ask you where you want to go eat or what movie you want to see and you respond, "Whatever you want; it doesn't matter to me"? There may indeed be times when you truly mean it. However, if you find yourself always saying this, chances are you're denying your own needs, at least some of the time, to keep the peace. Practice assertiveness by having an opinion and sticking to your decisions.

Owning Your Story

All of us have a story about how we got to where we are today. If we feel, in any way, that we're victims of our story and not owners of it, we will stay powerless. Personal victories and triumphs through adversity are usually a source of inspiration for others. People who aren't living in their personal power will use their stories as ways to get others to feel sorry for them or pity them for their circumstances. I once heard someone put it this way: "Your story did not happen to you; your story happened *for* you." When you are able to shift to this perspective, the world will open up to you. Your sense of empowerment will heal many aspects of your life.

At twenty-eight years old, I was diagnosed with thyroid cancer. I didn't let this news or experience define who I was or darken my view of life. I used it to create my new life and open myself to the possibility of helping others who are sick and suffering. While I struggled for a long time through my experience with cancer, I'm grateful for it because it made me the person I am today.

One of my favorite teachers, Dr. Wayne W. Dyer, used to say that life gives us lessons, and we can either get the lesson the first time, or we can repeat it. Owning our story but not living by it helps us get through to the lesson, learn from it, and move on.

I've also heard this lesson taught through the metaphor of

a diamond. Diamonds are formed in the Earth's upper mantle, about one hundred miles below the surface. Intense pressure and high temperatures form diamonds over time. They rise to the earth's surface by an intense explosive volcanic eruption that thrusts the diamonds upward at anywhere between twenty and thirty miles per hour. Diamonds that remain below the surface can't be appreciated or adored. A diamond's journey isn't easy, yet it's one of the most beautiful and rare gems on the planet. So it is for you. You won't shine as your most brilliant self without some pressure and heat. Every obstacle you encounter — every bit of criticism, letdown, or pushback — is designed to help you develop your sense of personal power.

Healing your emotional self in the third chakra is about appreciating all your life's circumstances not as forces against you but as forces for you, to propel you toward your highest self.

 ## Healing the Spiritual Body

Although the third chakra rests in the physical plane, there is something innately spiritual about its energy. In the second chakra we harness the power of creation, the creative force of the universe. To mold something new out of nothing is an incredible and miraculous power to behold. Yet creation for its own sake isn't all that fulfilling until it's presented to the world. When we shift from the second to the third chakra, we reveal our creation. Our creativity manifests in physical form, and we bring it to light. For example, the conception and nine-month growth of a baby isn't fulfilling to the parents in itself; only when the baby breaks out of the womb that has kept him protected and emerges into the world is he a complete joy for his creators.

WRITING DOWN YOUR INTENTIONS AND DESIRES

Your will and desires cannot manifest until you get clear on what you want out of life. You may meet people who are constant seekers, turning this way and that but lacking true direction. Solar energy is heating, penetrating, bright, and intense. If you're able to use this energy to create extreme focus, you can accomplish anything.

Have you ever walked into a dark room with a flashlight? If you shine the flashlight outward into the room, the light dissipates and covers a greater area. While it will give light, it's difficult to make out objects clearly. But if you focus the light on a specific object closer to you, you can examine the object in detail. Light is powerful. Focused and concentrated light, such as a laser, can cut through human flesh or even steel.

Setting your intentions and naming your desires is a way of focusing your energy and attention on a few things you would like to see manifested in your life. The act of focusing is half the work, as summed up in the expression "Where attention goes, energy flows."

Writing down your intentions and desires is a simple yet powerful process. There is no wrong way to do this. Get out a pen and paper or your favorite electronic device, and write down everything that comes to mind. Whatever you do, just get it out there. If it remains in your head, it's just an idea. Bring it out into the physical world. Don't worry about whether your desires are "realistic." The universe will handle those details. Intentions and desires that vibrate at a lower frequency won't manifest anyway. For example, if you write, "I'd like my mother-in-law to die," even if you're joking, that is a lower frequency desire, and it won't manifest. That being said, it might be worth exploring why you have those negative feelings toward her in the first place. But if you write down, "I'd like an

Audi convertible," that may or may not be a higher desire depending on its meaning in the overall trajectory of your life. In other words, try not to hold yourself back when writing this initial list of intentions and desires. See what comes up.

BEING HONEST WITH YOURSELF

When you're discovering who you are on the inside and who you wish to be on the outside, honesty is important. Many of us spend our entire lives trying to be what we think someone else wants us to be. We carefully select our words, behavior, and actions based on what others might think of us. It's impossible to harness your personal power if you succumb to masking your true self. Your job is to be the most authentic "you" you can be. Otherwise you will do a pretty awful job of being someone else — that isn't who you were designed to be. If you're someone who likes living with luxurious objects, don't pretend to be a monk. Or if you want to be single, don't get married simply to appease your family.

The third chakra is a good place to begin getting honest with yourself. Your intentions and desires list will give you the opportunity to see exactly where you are in your journey. For example, if you see a lot of material objects on your list, it could mean you're in a place where you don't feel that your financial or material needs are well met or you place great importance on status and position in the outer world. It might also indicate a lack of spirituality in your current life.

Honesty in this exercise isn't about judging yourself. It's about understanding where you are. And where you are is exactly where you're supposed to be. How can you change direction if you have no idea where you are?

When you get honest about who you are, you can break out of the mold. Let's go back to the analogy of the baby coming out of his mother's womb. Until he exits the womb and enters this world, and the cord is cut, he is completely and utterly dependent on his mother for everything. He cannot survive without her. Even after birth, for the first couple of years he must look to her for basic survival and nurturance. Then, as he grows, he begins to assert his independence and says, "Hey, world, this is who I am!" This assertiveness of will doesn't often come smoothly or easily. You may be all too familiar with the toddler's outbursts of willfulness: "I want to do this my way" or "I do it myself!" Such statements are examples of the child differentiating himself from his parents and caretakers and becoming an individual with wants, needs, and desires.

MANIPURA GUIDED MEDITATION

Sit or lie down comfortably with your spine elongated, and close your eyes. Breathe in deeply, allowing your lower belly to expand, and then exhale completely. Repeat twice. As you relax into your body, place your awareness on your solar plexus. Imagine a big circle surrounding your belly button like a bright shining sun. Then imagine a rotating disk moving through you, from your navel to your back on the other side. This spinning wheel is rotating and vibrating quickly as it generates open energy. Visualize the color yellow, vibrant like sunlight. Imagine the rays of this sun moving outward from your navel in all directions. This is your sense of personal power. This bright light is meant for you to shine outward into the world. It's the expression of your contribution to others through your gifts and talents. Fill yourself with the inner knowing that you can accomplish anything you set your mind to. You are powerful. You are strong. You have enormous passion and energy to achieve your goals.

As you bask in the glow of your personal power, bring to mind your intentions and desires. Like the sun that allows the planted seeds to fulfill their destiny, you know that your glowing solar energy gives life to your intentions and brings your desires toward their fulfillment. Your inner power breathes life into your intentions with each inhalation and exhalation. With time and patience you will bring the manifestation of your intentions to light. You know this to be true, and you have absolute confidence in yourself and your ability to manifest.

Feeling your third chakra energy, you know who you are. You have a strong sense of self. You are proud to show who you are to the world. You feel confident in your gifts, your talents, and what you have to offer. You can enhance the vibrations by chanting the mantra sound *RAM* three times.

Energy-Body Healing with Gems and Colors

Immersing yourself in solar energy, notably the sun, is the best way to heal through the color of the third chakra. If it's not sunny outside or it's a season when you don't see the sun much, spend time in the light of a full-spectrum sun therapy lamp.

Gemstones for the third chakra include amber, citrine, yellow tourmaline, and tiger's eye.

Third Chakra Mindfulness Ideas to Ponder

1. I can assert my will in a positive manner. I stand true to my beliefs and am entitled to my own opinion.
2. I am confident in who I am, and I own my story.
3. Honesty with myself and others is the only way to authenticity.
4. I am strong in my personal power, and I will take steps today to enhance my inner fire.

4 THE HEART CHAKRA
Anahata

ELEMENT: Air (Vayu)
COLOR: Emerald Green
MANTRA SOUND: *YUM*
SPECIAL HEART CHAKRA MANTRA:
Om mani padme hum

The fourth chakra is located in the heart center. It's where matter and spirit meet. It marks the halfway point, with three chakras below and three above. This is a very important chakra indeed, as it's our center of love and connection.

Here you transcend the confines of the lower chakras and move into a greater awareness of living in dharma, your righteous duty or virtuous path. Love flows from you. You are peaceful, joyful, and compassionate. Your actions are no longer self-serving but are motivated by helping others overcome suffering.

Anahata encompasses the heart center, lungs, arms, and hands. It also includes the circulatory and lymphatic systems.

The flow of prana, or life force, is prominent in the fourth chakra as the lungs reside here. Air flows in and out from the time you are born until the time you take your last breath. The strength of prana is regulated in part by control of the breath.

The mind, in turn, remains calm or becomes agitated based on your ability to regulate your breath. The slower and more controlled your breath becomes, the calmer your mind. A faster, erratic breathing pattern gives way to rapid, disorganized thought, which can lead to anxiety, panic, and even psychosis. A panic attack cannot manifest in the presence of a calm, even, and steady breath.

The Anahata chakra is also where your deepest heartfelt desires reside. While you have desires that emanate from the second and third chakras, fourth chakra desires are deeper and more profound, with a greater spiritual quality to them.

Two Ayurvedic doshas are predominant in the fourth chakra: Kapha and Vata. The main seat of the Kapha dosha is in and around the chest, including the stomach, lungs, heart, bronchial passages, and mucus membranes that line the respiratory system. Vata, too, has a main role in the fourth chakra as the chakra's element is air, one of the components of Vata. The sense of touch and the sense organ skin are both integral parts of the Vata dosha and the fourth chakra. Also, Vata's subdosha, *prana vata*, located in the heart and lungs, is responsible for the upward flow of air.

The gunas ruling the fourth chakra are rajas and sattva.

The color we attribute to the heart chakra is emerald green. The mantra, or bija (seed) sound, we vocalize for the fourth chakra is *YUM*.

Fourth Chakra Ailments

While imbalances in any of the chakras can create disease, those in the heart chakra can cause major, life-threatening diseases. Mind, body, and spirit are intimately linked, and the anatomical region of the heart chakra governs major life-sustaining bodily systems. Among them are respiration and heart health, which is why I encourage you to make certain that you keep the heart chakra open and aligned. In the United States, heart disease is the number one cause of death, and respiratory disease is the third.

Ailments of the fourth chakra include heart disease, lung disease, blood pressure issues, thymus problems, vascular problems, respiratory and circulatory problems, and breast problems such as breast cancer.

Fourth Chakra Energy

The English translation for the Sanskrit word *Anahata*, "unstruck" or "unhurt", embodies perfectly the energy of the fourth chakra. Love, the emotion of the fourth chakra, can be vague and difficult to understand in its fullest sense. You can say in the same thought, "I love chocolate and I love my mom," but love of those two things has different meanings. Loss of chocolate may not generate the same reaction as loss of your mother, yet you can use the same word to describe the emotion you feel about both things.

The fourth chakra bridges matter and spirit, and we begin to experience a more altruistic form of love that only grows with greater spiritual awareness. In the first three chakras, love is mostly motivated by having needs met. The first chakra meaning of love is "I love so I can get my needs met." Second chakra love is "I love so the other will love me back." Third chakra love is "I love so others can recognize I'm a good person and therefore I'm able to love myself." These are all stages of development in love and not inherently wrong, but they can be immature expressions of love.

Growing in spiritual maturity, when you reach the fourth

chakra, love comes from a less conditional source. You learn to love regardless of being hurt and regardless of whether others meet your needs all the time. You love because you know that, like honesty, learned in the third chakra, love is a higher vibrational frequency that will lead you to greater authenticity.

A young child being reprimanded will often say to her parent, "I hate you, Mommy! I hate you, Daddy!" A parent operating from the fourth chakra responds not with hatred but with love. The greatest spiritual leaders of the past always responded with love in the presence of hate. Jesus said to God while being crucified, "Father, forgive them, for they know not what they do." Mahatma Gandhi forgave those who oppressed him. Nelson Mandela forgave those who imprisoned him for twenty-seven years. These examples embody the true meaning of Anahata. Despite being hurt physically, mentally, and emotionally, they did not allow the hatred to penetrate their hearts.

A person in fourth chakra energy, who is "unstruck," experiences strikes from others but without the marks of being struck. That is powerful. Their sense of worth, well-being, and ability to love is no longer measured by external forces. The love from within radiates outward.

Our Societal Relationship with the Fourth Chakra

The form of love most often portrayed in the media is not the true form of love from the fourth chakra. But we do have moments when we touch on this love, often during times of crisis, when people make sacrifices to help others. For example, after Hurricane Harvey damaged 203,000 homes and caused $180 billion in damage, federal emergency workers rescued 10,000 people trapped under their homes or on the highways. American companies pledged over $157 million toward recovery efforts. A great number of other people poured money into charities such as the Red Cross to aid the rescue and recovery efforts. Outpourings of love often take the form of volunteerism for those in need, and these acts of selflessness are an expression of fourth chakra energy. However, on a societal level, the degree of consciousness doesn't consistently calibrate at the level of unconditional love.

To help you fully grasp the different levels of love, I'd like to share definitions of the word *love* from concepts in Greek philosophy. While there are around seven different definitions of love in Greek, I will present a handful to point out how our societal view of love relates to fourth chakra love.

Eros

Society today often defines love in the way of passion and sexual attraction. If you look at TV shows, movies, and advertising, the portrayal of love is about immediate satisfaction and passionate romance. Much of the draw to reality TV today is because of the display of eros and society's attraction to it. Eros mostly represents the first and second chakra energy of survival and procreation.

Philia

Deep friendship, brotherly bonds, and camaraderie all define the essence of philia. This type of love represents goodwill to others for a cause or purpose. Much of society is built upon this kind of love. For example, people who serve together in the armed forces have a special bond; those who attend the same schools, belong to the same fraternal organizations, or work for the same companies tend to get together for celebrations; and fans of the same sports teams bond with one another.

Philia bonds are formed through community and connection and are important for society as a whole, as having citizens who are lovingly connected is better than having isolated individuals who feel alone.

Philautia

Philautia, or self-love, can express itself negatively or positively. On the negative end, philautia can manifest as narcissism, with the person becoming self-obsessed and driven to acquire personal glory, fame, and power. The positive expression of philautia is when the person experiences self-love from a higher level of consciousness and shares that higher love with others. Self-love in the negative becomes a disservice to society as a whole.

While I am not skeptical in general, I do see a trend today of narcissism affecting society. Whether it's politicians seeking political power for their own self-glorification or young people seeking five thousand likes for selfie pictures, this "me only" worldview is dangerous. It creates an "us" versus "them" mentality that causes one group to rise up against another, and in the end, everyone gets hurt.

The negative form of philautia is the same as negative or unbalanced third chakra energy. It's when the unruly child is ruling the world.

Agape

The highest form of love and the one that best represents the fourth chakra is agape. This is an altruistic form of love. When the Greeks defined agape, it was in relation to God's love for us and our love for God. This kind of selfless love is extended to everyone, including strangers or enemies. As Pope Francis so eloquently voiced during the 2016 US presidential elections, love is about building bridges and not walls.

Agape is about realizing that when you help others, you are helping yourself. In the fourth chakra you begin to understand that there is no separation.

Society as a whole can make this shift in consciousness when enough individuals make the conscious choice to live at this level of love. Life is no longer about survival or getting what's "mine" but about going through life with the attitude "How can I help?" and "How can I serve?" When enough of us make this decision and it reaches critical mass, we can all move forward in a new direction to awaken to a different state of being.

Living Life in the Anahata Chakra

The transition from living life in the lower chakras to living life in the higher chakras is akin to awakening from a deep slumber for the first time. Life is no longer rooted in survival, procreation, attainment of worldly pleasures, pleasing others, or self-serving goals. Life now becomes an expression of service to others through compassion, giving, and openheartedness. Fourth chakra living doesn't embody the go-getter attitude of third chakra energy, but rather a passive openness, which attracts others to it. While the third chakra embodies yang, or masculine energy, the fourth chakra holds yin, or feminine energy. An air of peacefulness surrounds Fourth chakra people. They're lighthearted and laugh heartily. Their laughter is contagious. Love flows from their beings.

Fourth chakra people are compassionate to those around

them. Their hearts ache and feel deeply for those who suffer. Their sense of empathy is real. They readily cry or laugh with others out of genuine connection to their experiences. Their giving comes from kindheartedness and not from selfish motives. The light that radiates from their hearts attracts others to them.

I've had the great pleasure of meeting Mata Amritanandamayi, or as her followers affectionately call her, Amma. She's known as the "hugging saint." Besides running many charitable organizations, she goes around the world giving hugs to people for sometimes up to twenty-two hours per day, not leaving a site until everyone who wants a hug receives one. Amma grew up poor in southern India. Even as a child with little to no resources, Amma would give to others in need. According to her Hindu religion, suffering comes as a result of karma, or past action that must be repaid. In pondering this concept, Amma continually asks, "If it is one man's karma to suffer, isn't it our dharma (duty) to help ease his suffering and pain?" Amma truly represents fourth chakra love. As you sit in her presence, you can feel the peacefulness and calm that radiate from her being. Her eyes dance with joy and laughter. It's impossible to see any turmoil within her. Having felt her powerful vibrational energy, I can only imagine what being in the presence of Jesus must have been like. True love vibrates at a higher frequency than most of us can imagine.

Recognizing Fourth Chakra Imbalances

Vulnerability is an attribute of the fourth chakra. To experience the rewards that emanate from the heart requires openheartedness, a two-way exchange of giver and receiver in an authentic manner. Intimacy and closeness are the prizes to be gained by your willingness to be vulnerable.

The limitations arise in recognition that we don't live in a vacuum and that even those who live most of the time in fourth chakra energy also live in the energy of the first three chakras. If you've read the limitations of the first three chakras, you've also learned how they can easily bring you back down to lower states of consciousness.

I'm sure you've experienced moments of vulnerability at some point in your life. You opened your heart to someone and received hurt in exchange. Once this happens often enough, you learn to put up walls or close your heart to love altogether. The limitation lies in being selective in your willingness to love and be loved based on past experience.

Giving in to the fourth chakra limitations can lead to a continual fear of rejection and loneliness, and therefore putting up more walls. As you keep people out, those same people who once opened up to you and approached you with love will eventually leave, which further validates your fear of intimacy and vulnerability.

The way to end this cycle is to access higher sources of love that come from your spiritual connection to your Creator. Healing your heart each time you're afflicted by someone else or even by self-disappointment is crucial to not falling prey to fourth chakra limitations.

Maturity and growth in this chakra come from the realization that you don't need to remain in a state of hurt. You recognize that you have nothing to gain and everything to lose when you refuse openness.

Accepting Fourth Chakra Gifts

As many of us are used to the eros form of love, we become used to chaos and drama. We tend to associate true love and real-life experiences with a sense of disharmony that comes from passion. When we experience moments of peace and harmony, we can disregard them or brush them off as boring as we look for the next intense experience. Some people will even pick fights, find points to argue, or surround themselves with dramatic people just to "keep things interesting."

Being fully open to fourth chakra gifts is about being able to find peace in the midst of chaos. It's about letting go of drama in exchange for deeper enjoyment in the events of life. As I once heard Dr. Deepak Chopra say, "Where is the enjoyment in chaos and hysteria?" When you find your sense of inner peace, life begins to flow. You become lighthearted and you're able to laugh in any life circumstance. You're aware that there is beauty in all things, even in tragedy, and that beautiful things can be born out of tragedy. One example is Mothers Against Drunk Driving (MADD), which was formed in 1980 by moms who'd lost their children. This great organization has managed to lower the number of deaths by drunk and drugged drivers by 55 percent since its inception. I'm sure you're able to think of other organizations that were born as a result of tragic events.

Living in laughter, love, peace, and harmony daily doesn't mean you have to sit in a drum circle singing "Kumbaya" all day, and the world wouldn't necessarily benefit from that anyway. When you live from a space of inner peace, you automatically raise the consciousness of those around you, even as you go about the mundane activities of your day. You get in touch with a more spiritual existence in each moment. Your experiences become more meaningful as your perception widens.

Healing Anahata

DAILY AFFIRMATION

Om mani padme hum.
May the lotus flower contained within my heart
be open to love, compassion, and forgiveness.

 Healing the Physical Body

Cardiovascular exercise is one of the best things you can do for your physical health in the fourth chakra. Doing cardio every day is most important and can be achieved through brisk walking for thirty minutes daily. Of course, if you enjoy other cardio activities, you can mix up your routine, but strive for movement that will elevate your heart rate to between 50 and 85 percent of your maximum heart rate for at least thirty minutes at a time. As a member of a Western and mostly sedentary society, you will see enormous benefits when you add this simple routine to your day.

To prevent blockages in the heart and cardiac plexus, as well as to keep your respiratory health optimal, you can eat a mostly vegetarian diet with a heavy emphasis on leafy green vegetables, berries, whole grains, lentils, beans, herbs, and spices. Since the Ayurvedic Kapha dosha governs the area of the chest, a Kapha-pacifying diet is especially beneficial if you have heart disease, high blood pressure, or respiratory illnesses. You can learn more about all Ayurvedic diets in my first book, *The Wheel of Healing with Ayurveda: An Easy Guide to a Healthy Lifestyle.*

Yoga Asanas and Pranayama Exercises
to Heal the Fourth Chakra

All yoga breathing techniques are good for the fourth chakra, as each one enables you to breathe more fully. One simple breath I enjoy is what I call the four-count breath.

To view a video demo of these exercises, go to
www.youtube.com/c/MichelleFondinAuthor.
Click on the Playlists tab, and select
Chakra Healing Asanas & Pranayamas.
Scroll down the list until you find the one you're looking for.

Four-Count Breath: Sit with your spine tall, and roll your shoulders back and down. With your lips closed, begin inhaling through your nose as you inflate your lower belly. Inhale to the count of four. Then hold your breath for four counts and exhale through your nose for four. Repeat this breath for two to five minutes. As you become more accustomed to breathing in this way, you can increase the count to five, six, or seven.

Thymus Thump: The thymus gland is located at the center of the chest below the collarbone. It is an important gland for the immune system and is particularly large during childhood, when it produces most of the body's T-cells, an extremely important type of white blood cell that protects us from pathogens. The thymus shrinks in adulthood and its function diminishes. You can strengthen your immune system and your energy level by practicing the thymus thump, which looks exactly like Tarzan thumping his chest.

Make fists with both your hands, and place them against the center of your chest, a few inches apart from each other, with your knuckles about three finger-widths below your collarbone. As you inhale, pound on the center of your chest, alternating between your two fists. Exhale the word *ah* while you continue thumping. Repeat the exercise for four complete breaths.

Cow Face Pose — *Gomukhasana*: Sit on a yoga mat with your knees bent and your feet flat on the mat. Draw your left foot inward and set it down on the mat underneath your right leg close to your right hip. Then bring your right leg over the top, and set your right foot down on the mat close to your left hip. Your knees should be aligned in the middle, with the right one on top of the left. If you're unable to fold your legs in this manner, sit in a simple cross-legged position. Reach your left arm out to the left. Bend the arm downward and fold it behind your back with your fingers reaching upward. Bring your right arm straight up in the air and then fold it behind your head and reach for your left hand. If you're able, clasp your hands together behind your back. If you can't reach, hold on to a scarf, necktie, or yoga strap, with one end in each hand, and walk your hands as close to each other as possible. Once you've clasped your hands together, lengthen through the spine and keep your head in a neutral position. Breathe deeply from your lower belly, and hold the pose for five breaths. Switch to the other side and repeat the exercise. Cow face pose opens the chest and stimulates the lymphatic system.

Camel Pose — *Ustrasana*: While camel pose is wonderful for opening the area of the heart and cultivating the fourth chakra attribute of vulnerability, it can be quite challenging for a yoga beginner. Gather the following props if you're new to yoga or unfamiliar with this pose: a folded blanket or towel and two yoga blocks. (If you don't have yoga blocks, you can use two stacks of books, both roughly even in height, about nine inches tall.)

Start by kneeling on your yoga mat with your knees hip-width apart and with one block at its maximum height next to each of your feet. If your knees are sensitive, place the folded blanket underneath your knees. Either rest the tops of your feet on the mat or flex your toes and tuck them under, depending on your comfort level with leaning on flexed feet. With your hips directly above your knees, lengthen your spine upward and then arc it backward toward your feet. Bring your hands behind you to hold on to your heels. If you can't reach your heels, rest one hand on each of the blocks. As you hold on to your heels or blocks, bring your pelvis forward and allow your head to extend backward and down toward the floor. If this causes discomfort in your neck, bring your chin down toward your chest instead. Hold the pose as long as you can while maintaining a steady, smooth breath. When you're finished, take child's pose (*balasana*) as a counterpose: lower your hips to the floor and then extend your torso forward and rest it between your thighs, with your forehead on the floor.

Standing Bow Pose — *Dandayamana Dhanurasana*: Stand on your mat with your feet together. Rest your gaze on a fixed point on the wall in front of you. This will be your focal point, or *drishti*. Lift your right foot behind you, and clasp your foot or ankle with your right hand either from the outside or the inside. If you hold your ankle, you will have a firmer grasp. If you can't quite catch your foot, you can use a yoga strap to hold it. Once you have your foot, reach your left arm forward in front of you, with your thumb up and your fingers pointing forward. Lift up through the crown of your head, and press your foot or ankle into your hand as you lift the leg higher. Your torso will automatically come slightly forward as you create a bow shape with your right arm and leg. Balance comes from the dynamic of your left arm reaching forward as your right foot presses back against your right hand. Hold the pose for at least five breaths. Repeat on the other side.

 ## Healing the Emotional and Energetic Body

Healing the emotional body in the fourth chakra is by far one of the most important things you can do for your health. With years of experience in Ayurvedic lifestyle counseling, I am convinced that heart health is directly linked to our emotional state.

A few years ago I had a client come in for an Ayurvedic consultation. He had suffered a heart attack at age forty-five and had a stent put in. He wanted to learn how to manage stress and adopt a healthier lifestyle. During the consultation I asked him what had happened emotionally in his recent past. He looked at me strangely but answered that he couldn't think of anything except that he had gotten a divorce a couple of years prior to the heart attack. I shared with him that the divorce was likely a contributing factor to the heart attack. He wasn't convinced because he was only focused on the physical.

This is but one example. When there are blockages in the heart chakra, there is always an emotional component. Healing the heart — one of the most difficult things to do, yet crucial for growth — is mostly about letting go of past hurt and learning how to forgive.

LETTING GO OF PAST HURT

You don't always consciously choose what happens to you throughout life. You can't control how others will act around you or toward you. You can't even regulate another person's opinion of you. As long as there are people in your life, you can guarantee you will be emotionally hurt at some point. It's inevitable.

You're going through life trying to get your needs met, and so is everyone else. If I'm trying to get my needs met and you're trying to get your needs met, there will be some clashes. Most of the time when someone hurts you or disagrees with you, it's not even about you. Think about this for a second. Have you ever considered the idea that most people are absorbed with their own needs and desires?

The alcoholic father who ignores you is just worried about getting his next drink. The teacher who scolds you for talking is just trying to manage the thirty children in her class and to get the job done. The person who cuts you off on the road is just trying to get to work on time. The jealous sister who talks badly about you is just trying to get the attention and love that she feels she isn't receiving. Most of the time you're just in the way of another person getting his or her needs met. It doesn't make it right, just, or fair; it just is. Each person has his or her own pathway.

When you hold on to past hurt, you are weighing yourself down unnecessarily. You're creating heaviness in your own heart that could otherwise be lifted by simply letting go. Whatever happened in your past needed to happen so that you could be where you are today. If you had only good times or people who lifted you up all the time, you couldn't have had the emotional and spiritual growth to reach higher heights. You needed the adversity, resistance, and sometimes even hatred to propel you toward your destiny.

A couple of years back when I was training for a half marathon, I hired a personal trainer to teach me how to gain strength through weight training. I wanted to make sure I didn't injure myself, and I knew that by creating muscle mass I would be less prone to injury. During the first session the trainer worked me hard but took it a little easy on me. But after the first session he pushed me to the limit. He added more weight, created more resistance, and added even more repetitions. During the session, it was awful. I'm not good at handling pain. I complained and nearly cried, but I did what he asked me because I knew I wanted to be stronger. You might argue that I was paying him to put me through this adversity. While this is true, I couldn't have gained muscle mass without the pain and resistance. I was hurting after every session, to the point of barely being able to walk the next day. But I was grateful, because I knew that the next time I encountered his tough workouts it would be easier, for a time. If I had avoided the workouts and the weight lifting I wouldn't have seen any positive changes in my body.

Letting go of past hurt is as easy as a decision. Your ego might tell you otherwise, but it's really that simple. Yes, you may have grown up in an abusive household. You may have had a spouse cheat on you. Any number of things may have happened in your past, however unfortunate. Yet the choice to hold on to the hurt or to let it go is all yours.

When you make the choice to let go, it doesn't mean continuing to put yourself in the same situations that allowed the hurt in the first place. It means letting go and then making different choices that can put you on a different path.

FORGIVENESS

Once you make the conscious choice to release the hurt and pain, the only way to completely heal your heart is through the power of forgiveness. The act of forgiveness is extending grace to a person (including yourself) for what occurred. Offering forgiveness doesn't mean you're condoning the act itself or suggesting that it was acceptable. Forgiveness means that

you're choosing peace rather than the turmoil that the grievance holds. When you hold on to the need to be right or to
seek revenge in any way, you're destroying your own heart. The
other person has perhaps long forgotten what happened. Or
maybe the person never realized she'd done anything wrong in
the first place. By keeping the grievance alive in your heart, you
are allowing the poison to grow.

I once had a client whose husband had committed suicide
five years prior to our conversation. Even though they were
separated when he took his life, she confessed that she was still
furious at him for selfishly killing himself, as they had a young
daughter who needed him. I explained to her that by holding
that anger she wasn't hurting him (he was already dead), but
she was hurting herself. I suggested that she write him a letter
outlining all the reasons why she was angry, after which she was
to place it on his grave or burn it to let go of all the negativity.

Letting go of hurt and forgiving are about keeping your
heart space pure.

 Healing the Spiritual Body

When man has love, he is no longer at the mercy of forces greater
than himself, for he, himself, becomes the powerful force.
— LEO BUSCAGLIA

The most important lesson we can learn from our emerging
spirituality at the level of the fourth chakra is that our Creator
is infinite love. The wellspring of love flowing through the entire universe is infinite. There is no shortage of unconditional
love. Every person has equal access to this love regardless of
age, gender, race, or socioeconomic status. The question remains: How open are you to receiving this love?

Human love is almost always conditional in at least one aspect or another. If you expect perfect, unconditional love from another human being you will constantly be disappointed. The only perfect love is one that comes from your spiritual Source.

The awakening you experience in the fourth through seventh chakras is through harnessing this unconditional love, from your Source, and being able to use it in your interactions and relationships. In order to best achieve this, you will need to regularly practice balancing through letting go of the constant demands of the ego.

Those demands sound something like this:

"I don't want to forgive him. He started it."

"She hurt me first when I was being nice."

"He doesn't deserve a second chance."

"She ruined my life with her betrayal."

"I hate him."

As I mentioned in the third chakra, you will never lose your ego completely while you are alive. You can, however, hush it down a bit. This generally happens when you shift your internal conversation from "What's in it for me?" to "What's in it for you?"

Choosing Peace

The ego is always concerned about being hurt, affronted, and humiliated. It's constantly in reaction mode. Dr. Wayne W. Dyer used to quote frequently from *A Course in Miracles*: "I can choose peace rather than this." When you're confronted with expressions of hatred and fear, you can choose how you react to them. You can react with your ego or with your heart. It's a simple choice. It's not always easy to choose peace, but it's a choice nonetheless. And you will be continually confronted with people who will give you opportunities to practice. There is no shortage of these people.

Choosing peace might mean you walk away with no comment. It might mean you answer with empathy and understanding. Or it could mean you no longer wish to associate with that person. Choosing peace means making the choice not to be offended or to let other people's remarks harm you.

OPENING YOUR HEART

Cleansing your heart space is the first half of clearing the fourth chakra. The next part is keeping the doors to your heart open. In his book *Love: What Life Is All About*, psychologist Leo Buscaglia states, "Love is always open arms. If you close your arms about love, you will find that you are left holding only yourself." I believe this to mean that you should neither clasp too tightly nor release and then refuse to let anyone else in. When you love fully and unconditionally, your loved ones feel equally loved by you whether they are close or far, or whether they are pleasing you or not. Either way, it's all the same. The idea is to love in the same way that your Creator loves. God doesn't change his mind about the way he loves you. You have free will to come and go as you please. He will love you if you seek a relationship with him, and he'll love you if you don't. You have been given a choice. But he'll love you all the same.

Too often we set limits on love. We say things such as "I've opened my heart too much" or "I've given too much, and look where it's gotten me." Remember, every time you think of reasons not to open your heart to love, that is your ego getting in the way again.

PRACTICING COMPASSION

Merriam-Webster defines *compassion* as a "sympathetic consciousness of others' distress together with a desire to alleviate it." While the third chakra ego is much concerned with "me," "mine," and "Where am I going?" the fourth chakra spiritual essence revolves around the suffering of the world and how to end it. When your heart is moved by a touching story and you feel empathy for another, you're practicing compassion. When you reach in your pocket to give a dollar to a homeless person, you're allowing the spirit of compassion to enter your heart. Some people are naturally compassionate, while others aren't. I believe that compassion can be a learned trait.

One spring during Lent while I was living in France, I decided to take on a project that created a lot of discomfort in me. I wanted to do something good for others during the forty days prior to Easter instead of the traditional practice of giving up chocolate or sweets. In Aix-en-Provence, France, near where I lived, there were a lot of homeless people. Most of them were illegal immigrants, or gypsies, as the French called them. I made the decision to pack lunches every Wednesday during Lent and to go seek out homeless individuals in the city and give them the bagged lunches. In addition, I decided to take my three-year-old son with me. Coming from suburbia in the United States, I wasn't accustomed to homeless people or comfortable around them. I made the decision to put myself into discomfort to help other people. I didn't feel it was enough to give money or donate to a food bank. I needed to be on the streets and spontaneously giving and interacting with those less fortunate than I. It was the best thing, I believe, and the most difficult thing I've ever done.

At first, the homeless people I encountered were very

skeptical of my kindness. The French, in general, don't have a habit of taking kindly to homeless people. They have social systems in place that can give even a homeless person a monthly source of income. However, as I mentioned, most of these people were illegal immigrants and therefore not eligible to receive such aid. In the beginning I had to urge some of the homeless people to accept my lunches, especially those with children. But as time went on, they received me with open arms. I adapted to make extra for the homeless children with their parents or to include a little toy or plush animal. Seeing them would usually bring me to tears. Some Wednesdays I would get nervous because I didn't want to go out there and face them. Other times the weather was bad and I just didn't want to get out of my comfort zone to fulfill the promise I had made to myself and God. But I did. The level of compassion I achieved during that project was unmatched by anything else I've experienced. I believe the reason I was able to achieve that level, at that moment, was because I pushed myself to the edge of discomfort. I learned: the greater the self-sacrifice, the greater the inner reward.

I don't mention this story to pat myself on the back. Except for my family, most people have no idea I ever did this. I tell this story to demonstrate that you can heal your heart through acts of compassion. It doesn't have to be as big as making lunches for the homeless. You can offer someone a smile, a joke, or a warm hug. You can give a person the gift of your full attention by turning off your phone when you're with him or her. If you know your friend or family member has had a rough day, you can ask, "Is there anything I can do for you?" Then do it.

Awareness of others' suffering and a desire to alleviate their pain are all it takes.

ANAHATA GUIDED MEDITATION

Sit comfortably and close your eyes. Bring your awareness to your heart center, your source of love and compassion. Imagine, think, or feel an emerald green color
radiating from your heart. This sparkling green light is
shining outward in every direction. Breathe into this
space, and feel the circumference of the light surrounding your heart getting wider and wider. Feel the balance
between physical matter and spirit here. Feel yourself grounded and open and awakened to spirit at the
same time.

Now that you're aware of your radiating, compassionate light moving out of your body and into the
world, bring your attention back to your heart center.
Search within your heart for any discomfort that resides
there. If you find any, send the discomfort flowers and
then escort it away from your heart. As you're escorting
away the discomfort, which can come disguised as hurt,
shame, blame, anger, or lack of forgiveness, thank it for
its message and let it know that it can go now. Repeat
this with every source of discomfort that comes up in
your heart center, until you're only left with light and
ease of breath. You will know when you have let everything go because your heart will feel lighter, as if a large
weight has been lifted off your chest. Feel how easy it is
to breathe now.

Now that your heart is clear, feel flooded with unconditional love. Allow this love to flow in and fill your
heart space. Feel the warmth and expansiveness of this
love. Allow yourself to receive. Allow yourself to feel

vulnerable and open to this great love, of which you are worthy. You are becoming a vessel of love with each and every breath. Love flows to you and through you. You become a conduit for this love, and as this love fills every cell of your body, you feel lighter and more joyful. Your joyfulness radiates throughout your being. You may even find yourself smiling for no apparent reason. Let it be as it is, for this is the state of love. At this moment you may even feel a tingling sensation pulsating through your body. This is normal, as you have raised the vibrational frequency of your being. Sit with this sensation. It's here, and you can always access it whenever you desire.

You can sit in this silent meditation for as long as you like before opening your eyes and slowly returning to activity. To enhance the vibrations, chant the mantra sound *YUM* three times.

Energy-Body Healing with Gems and Colors

As mentioned earlier, the color for the fourth chakra is emerald green. You can wear this color or keep it in your awareness while healing your heart.

Rose quartz is the most beautiful and effective stone for bringing love and compassion into your life. Keep a rose quartz stone with you throughout the day. If you can, wear the stone close to your heart. You can even get a rose quartz in the shape of a heart to remind you of healing each time you hold it.

Fourth Chakra Mindfulness Ideas to Ponder

1. I am ready to release hurt from my heart and forgive everyone who has harmed me, including myself.
2. I am open to giving and receiving love and know I am worthy of love.
3. I feel compassion toward others, especially those whom I don't understand.
4. I am a vessel of God's love, transporting unconditional acceptance to all who need it.

5 THE THROAT CHAKRA
Vishuddha

ELEMENT: Space (Akasha)
COLOR: Sky Blue
MANTRA SOUND: *HUM*

The fifth chakra, which is the first chakra totally on the spiritual plane, is located in the throat and governs communication and creative verbal expression such as singing, chanting, reading poetry out loud, and recitation. When the fifth chakra is illuminated, all the lower chakras transcend their limitations.

The anatomical region of the fifth chakra includes the throat, neck, shoulders, thyroid, parathyroid, mouth, tongue, jaw, larynx, and vocal cords. The sense is hearing, and the sense organs are the ears.

The Sanskrit word *Vishuddha* means "purity," and I love this translation because it captures the true essence of the fifth chakra. Its purity comes from speaking the truth that resides in our hearts.

Pure means uncontaminated, clear, innocent, clean, or impeccable. When you reach this level of consciousness, you are exploring the part of you that is pure. You have reached the level of spirit that is unadulterated. From the heart chakra you come to a place where you are awakened to truth. That is such a beautiful realization. All the debris has been swept aside. In the lower chakras you had to sift through such debris to see the truth in everything. Now the only thing you see is truth, and it feels clear. There is liberation in seeing truth.

Vishuddha is like looking into the Caribbean Sea and not seeing the bottom of it. One year I took a trip to Jamaica. I had always seen pictures of the Caribbean with its crystal-clear turquoise waters and its white sands as far as the eye can see. When I arrived in Jamaica I didn't see what I had imagined. Around my hotel all I could see was lots of seaweed, rocks, and sand. I was so disappointed because I wanted to experience the beauty of the clear waters like I had seen in the pictures. In order to see this, I had to travel far by bus to find it. When I arrived, it was well worth the trip.

You have traveled up four chakras to find the clarity of the fifth. The debris of deception, lies, and confusion has drifted away, and you never again have to live in darkness.

The Ayurvedic dosha that rules the fifth chakra is Vata. The two gunas that rule this chakra are rajas and sattva.

The color we attribute to the throat chakra is cerulean blue. The mantra, or bija (seed) sound, we vocalize for the fifth chakra is *HUM*.

Fifth Chakra Ailments

Ailments of the fifth chakra include diseases of the throat and the thyroid and parathyroid glands, neck and jaw problems, speech impediments, colds, and hearing problems. From a psychological standpoint, imbalances can include unexpressed grief, sadness, anger, judgment, and feelings of depression.

Fifth Chakra Energy

The power that lies within the fifth chakra is the power to transcend space-time. Communication enables us to transcend space as sound waves travel through phone lines, cell towers, and internet connections. We can be virtually present in another place — through audio and more recently through video — without leaving our physical location.

Communication happens on many levels, not only the physical. We communicate through words and sounds, facial expressions, body language, thoughts (also known as telepathy), and vibration. A thought is a vibration on a subtle level, which will be explained in more detail in the chapter on the sixth chakra. The organs and body parts in the fifth chakra allow us to create and absorb the vibrations of sound.

Sound can be used to harm or to heal. The voice of a loved one can be used to say, "I love you," or it can be used to say, "I never want to see you again." When used for unkind intentions, such as in rap lyrics filled with words of hate, sound creates separateness and dissonance. However, when harnessed as a powerful expression of beauty, as in Mozart's Forty-First Symphony or Beethoven's Fifth, it creates harmony, entrainment, and synchronization.

Words have the power to heal when you speak inner truth to yourself. Your inner and outer dialogue about yourself determines how healthy you are. If you repeat to yourself daily, "I'm so fat and I'll never get thin," those words have the power to become your reality. However, if you tell yourself, "I'm working on getting healthier each and every day," you will have quite a different outcome. Words from others also have the power to heal. When a child falls and skins his knee, he will heal faster if his parent says, "You're all right. Get up and go play."

When I was in France around 2006, I went to the eye doctor

because I was having trouble reading. I was thirty-five years old at the time and thought my age was contributing to the fuzzy words I was seeing. I shared this thought with the doctor, who told me it had nothing to do with age and that I had some sort of eye disease that would cause me to need stronger and stronger prescriptions as the years went on. He was very elaborate as he spoke about my future with certainty and conviction. I was taken aback that he, a medical doctor, could "read" into my future and dared say so with such doom and gloom. Luckily, I was already on a spiritual path of knowing that we create our own destiny, so I brushed it off as ignorance. However, his words did have power because I remember them to this day. Now at age forty-six, eleven years later, my sight isn't a whole lot worse. My prescription has changed once, but I'm optimistic about my vision staying the same or getting better over the next decade or more.

Can you see the potential damage in the words you or others speak? Had I believed the doctor and taken his words to be reality, I probably would be blind by now. His words were not truth, but a potential truth.

On the positive side of words, have you noticed that when you talk to a person you're close to, your speech patterns tend to mimic each other's? Words connect in fluid harmony people who like to be together. You can notice this best in teenagers. Listen to the way they speak. They create their own language with words that only they seem to understand. If you have a teenager, you know this. And the language changes quickly, every few years or so. Words such as *sick* to describe something awesome or *LOL*, taken from text-speak to mean "laugh out loud," are already outdated, according to my teenager, when his siblings used those words only four years ago.

Singing and chanting are ageless forms of sound vibration.

Singing has been used for thousands of years to band people together with a purpose. Song has the power to transcend. Much of today's soul music originated from music sung by enslaved Africans in the Americas. They used songs to strengthen community and transcend the conditions in which they were living. They also used song to connect with God, which brought them to a state of transcendent bliss.

Singing and chanting can be used unconsciously for brainwave entrainment. People with close relationships entrain, which means their bodily rhythms work together in synchronistic harmony through sound. Mothers chant or sing to their babies to soothe their cries. When my children were babies and they were fussy or I was trying to get them to sleep, I used to hum a simple, repetitive tune to them. I'm not sure if I spontaneously made it up or if perhaps it was hummed to me when I was a baby. I only hummed it to each of them for their first year of life or so, when babies need the most soothing. The strange thing is, the other day my youngest son, who is now thirteen, told me of the tune I hummed to him as a baby. He hummed it back to me and said, "Mom, I loved it when you hummed that tune to me. I remember it well." He couldn't have been more than a year old when he last heard it, being that he is the youngest. How could he remember it now, twelve years later? I believe the power of that sound created synchronization in his brain that signaled well-being. So now as a young man, when he has a sense of well-being, in particular around me as his mother, that sound comes to mind as one of his earliest memories of well-being.

You too can entrain your cells to work in synchronistic harmony through sound. In each chapter, I provide a mantra sound you can use for chanting. By chanting the sound *HUM* repeatedly, you will align the vibrational energy in the fifth chakra and cause your cells to remember their purpose and work toward the greater good, which in this case is keeping you healthy and whole. Mantras in meditation are used for this purpose too. You can chant a mantra, incantation, or affirmation out loud or even in your mind, and it will have the same effect. Simple, primordial mantras chanted out loud have greater vibrations and therefore have greater power. For example, chanting the sound *OM*, while allowing your lips to vibrate on the *mmmmm* sound as you exhale, creates an explosion of vibrations in the body and precipitates healing. Chanting out loud the affirmation "I am strong, I am healthy" has great power too, just in a different way with different intensity.

The ultimate healing power in the Vishuddha chakra enables you to synchronize communication between your inner and outer worlds and most importantly to clear the lines of communication to the Divine. Once you have harnessed this power, wherein there is no disconnection or disharmony in communication between you, others, and the Divine, you will have a clear path toward enlightenment.

The first step toward this path is to seek and speak truth.

Our Societal Relationship with the Fifth Chakra

Truthfulness has become more difficult than ever in modern society. We have increased means of communication, and we seemingly communicate all the time. With the constant stream of text messages, voicemails, video calls, social media feeds, and emails, it appears that we're communicating at a more constant rate than at any other time in history. And perhaps we are.

Yet much of this communication — such as humble-brag Facebook posts or tweets — is one-way and often designed to embellish or conceal the truth. I'm not suggesting that people are inherently dishonest. I don't have such a bleak outlook on people's subconscious intentions. However, that faceless and often voiceless communication can result in a portrayal of an alternate reality.

With in-person communication, you can also alter the other person's perception of who you are by filtering what you let them see. But when you're face-to-face with another, you have other cues to send you signals as to whether the person is sincere. You can "read" a person's energy field (we all do this whether consciously or unconsciously). You can notice a person's body language. You can connect intonation of voice with facial expressions. It's much more difficult to deceive in person than over the internet or the phone.

Today, much of the political climate in the United States is a result of modern society's one-way communication through declarative statements, insults, or proclamations of reality without any instant return of communication by the receiving parties. The term *alternative facts*, coined in 2017 by the Trump administration, demonstrates the tendency to ignore truth in favor of the alternate world of the internet in which truth doesn't seem to be valued by all.

When I was on the internet dating scene, I was astonished to discover how much people lied in their profiles. There seems to be a cultural tolerance of "acceptable untruths" (or blatant lies, as I call them) in things such as dating profiles and even résumés. It's rather humorous if you think about it, because we have greater access to truth today. In the past, if you wanted to fact-check a given topic, you really had to search. Fact-checking often meant trips to the library and in-person research at various locations. Today we can search facts instantly. Yet it seems that many people don't want to see the truth.

Society will only shift to a perception of truthfulness as an asset and a necessity when enough people decide that it must be so.

Another issue with communication today has to do with the expectation of a rapid response. Because we're used to instantaneous feedback through instant messaging or texts, we're inclined to become impatient when we don't receive a response right away. Two things tend to happen in these situations: (1) we jump the gun and respond harshly when we don't get an instant response, and (2) the person on the other end may answer with a less-than-honest, ill-conceived, or poorly researched response because he or she is more concerned with answering quickly than with thinking things through first.

The same happens with our listening skills. Fifth chakra energy is as much about hearing and listening as speaking. Both sides are equally important for effective communication. Through all our electronic ways of communicating, we have become accustomed to jumping to conclusions and laying out what we want to say without necessarily taking in what the other person is saying. Then it becomes two one-sided pieces of communication that never merge into a conversation.

One way to rectify this imbalance is to realize that communication is a dynamic dance of giving and receiving that operates according to a patterned rhythm. If you're blurting out nonstop whatever comes to mind over various forms of media, you aren't honoring the natural rhythm of this dance. By taking the time to truly listen to what the other person is saying and asking questions when you aren't sure or don't understand, you can help turn the tide back toward authentic and real communication.

Another pitfall of using electronic communication is that it can let barriers down inappropriately. Cyberpsychologists have noticed a dramatic increase in behavior traditionally reserved for those under the influence of alcohol or drugs, that of dropping all defenses and blurting out the truth. People who have had a few drinks tend to lose their inhibitions and tell all or "tell it like it is." The same phenomenon can happen when we're hiding behind a username or social media profile. Our typical inhibitions, including a healthy dose of caution, seem to fade away too easily. Many open themselves up to complete strangers, feeling safe when they see reciprocation of such behavior. This lack of discernment in communication can be just as dangerous as its opposite: completely shutting down communication closes off the fifth chakra, but throwing it all out there online or in dialogues with people on the internet whom you haven't met in person can push you into a deceptive reality. In real life and in healthy communication, the give-and-take allows the two parties to open up gradually. Going back to the online dating example, one of the dating websites I was on years ago had an entire page on online dating etiquette, and I found it responsible and helpful. A couple of pieces of advice stuck out in particular, and I remember them to this day. The first is, communication is give-and-take. If you initiate communication, wait for the other person to respond. It's a back-and-forth effort. Try not to dominate the conversation. The second piece of advice was a warning of what we're exploring in this section: if a person is opening themselves up too quickly and acting as if they're falling in love straightaway, that should be a warning sign to get away quickly.

I believe the lesson we can take away from our societal relationship with the fifth chakra is that a multifaceted approach to communication is necessary to foster healthy and honest relationships. Meeting in person is more important than a phone call or an electronic message. Remember to listen and actually hear what the other person is saying, as well as get your message across. Use the tool of asking questions and repeating back to make sure you heard properly what the other person is saying. Finally, remember that immediacy of response is not always the healthiest or for the highest good of both parties. At times, thoughtful reflection can help you and the other person get in touch with your highest truth.

Living Life in the Vishuddha Chakra

The ruling planet of the fifth chakra is the planet Jupiter. The Sanskrit word for *Jupiter* is *guru*, which means "dispeller of darkness." Therefore, people who embody fifth chakra energy enlighten others with their speech and words. Fifth chakra people have transcended their egos in such a way that they're in touch with their souls. They become seekers and speakers of truth. They have spent time in their heart chakra and have opened their hearts to higher spiritual knowledge. When they speak or write, they're inspired and, in turn, inspire others. Their voices are melodious and welcomed by those who want to learn these truths.

Recognizing Fifth Chakra Imbalances

Signs that the fifth chakra is out of balance may include the Vata imbalance of talking incessantly without listening. This kind of nervous talking uses the voice out of fear of silence or fear of being alone. Another manifestation of imbalance would be using the voice to be harsh to others, such as putting a person in his or her place or being overly critical. Those out of balance can also use their voice as a weapon to hurt another person by not speaking or by yelling, screaming, or crying out loud to create drama.

Speech impediments are disorders that can limit your voice or cause frustration in speaking. A person who feels suppressed and doesn't feel he or she has a voice can experience blockages in the fifth chakra.

Miscommunication and misunderstandings are also limitations of the fifth chakra. This often happens when two people are talking at each other rather than to each other, and when one person isn't listening or doesn't understand.

Take care not to misdirect your fifth chakra energy by using your newly acquired spiritual knowledge to try to convince others of your perspective. Maybe you know people who have done this with you, talking nonstop and shoving their perspective down your throat. Instead of speaking to convince, balanced fifth chakra people speak to inspire. Think of a speaker who has inspired you. Those with inspiration, which means "in spirit," will usually talk about themselves in order to demonstrate their path toward enlightenment. It's never about "You should do this or that" but rather "This is what I did and what I experienced." That leaves you the space to have an aha moment. Space, akasha, which is the element of the fifth chakra, is the essential component in verbal expression. I once heard that it's not the words in the books that make beautiful stories but the spaces in between; and it's not the musical notes that create sweet melodies but the pauses in between those notes. It's about space.

In the preface I mentioned having to heal my fifth chakra energy after my thyroid cancer surgery. To that end, I had to do a lot of self-reflection on how this energy had developed throughout my childhood. I'm the firstborn, and when I was five my parents divorced. However, the divorce is not my earliest memory. I have lots of memories, from as early as age three, of my parents fighting and my mom crying. I even remember giving my mom boxes of Kleenex. Through this traumatic experience, I believe I developed a habit of "being good" and not creating waves. My mom would even tell me that I was her strength. Since I had to take care of my mother's emotions and look after my sister, I developed an inner notion that my own feelings weren't as important. In order to heal, I had to learn to express myself. It didn't come easily. And at times when I tried to make my voice heard, it came out as shouting. But over time I learned to be more assertive and not bottle up my feelings.

Accepting Fifth Chakra Gifts

In free societies we take for granted the gifts of speaking and hearing truth. The fact that we have ears to listen and a mouth to speak is a miracle in itself. Understanding language, being able to read and write, and the gift of communication wonderfully bond us together on a deeper level than only the physical.

Being able to freely express ourselves without fear of being persecuted for our opinions, political views, or religious persuasions is a gift. I recently ran a half marathon in Washington, DC. There were spectators holding inspirational signs to help the runners keep running. Some of the signs read "If Trump can run and win, so can you" and "You can run better than the government." I thought, *How fortunate we are to live in a place where this freedom of expression exists!* In another country those spectators with signs might be arrested. If you're a female or a minority in some countries, you cannot speak your mind, vote, or even drive.

Your inner truth and voice are powerful blessings to use whenever you can.

Healing Vishuddha

DAILY AFFIRMATION

I can easily speak my inner truth.

 Healing the Physical Body

In order to effectively speak your truth, your throat, vocal cords, mouth, jaw, and hearing must remain healthy. Eating the wrong foods and maintaining poor posture can contribute to ineffective vocal expression. If you find speaking, singing, chanting, or projecting your voice to be challenging, the following changes may help.

First, dry mouth can be rectified by reducing caffeine and alcohol consumption and by decreasing the number of dry foods in your diet such as crackers, chips, dried fruit, and nuts. You can also keep your mouth moist and throat lubricated by swishing and gargling daily with an organic food-grade sesame oil. Take one to two teaspoons in your mouth and swish for one minute, then gargle lightly and spit it out. It will leave a light film in your mouth. You can do this before bed and you will reap the benefits of a lubricated mouth and the antibacterial effects of the sesame oil. Phlegm in your throat can be corrected by reducing cold dairy, sugar, and processed foods.

Next, sitting at a desk and staring at a computer all day can cause poor posture due to craning the neck forward to see the screen. Whenever you notice yourself in this position, make a correction: sit straight, and draw your head and shoulders back to bring your spine into better alignment.

CHANTING AND SINGING

Saying the chakra mantra sounds or other mantras out loud is great for toning the throat and strengthening the vocal cords. Singing brings about joy and can be transcendent. It's no wonder so many of us sing in the shower or alone in the car. It brings out a side of us that is often hidden. Liberate your fifth chakra energy by singing out loud — not only in the shower or car.

HEAD AND NECK EXERCISES

Because we tend to position the neck improperly when using electronic devices, it's very important that we stretch our necks frequently to release the tired muscles.

Sit tall with your back straight. Have your head in a neutral position with your chin neither up nor down. Rest your hands on your lap with your palms facing up. Turn your head to the right, then bring your chin down and draw a semicircle with your chin as you bring it to your left. Then bring your chin downward from the left side and draw a semicircle back to the right. Continue back and forth eight times. Next, return your head back to a centered, neutral position. Take the first two fingers of your right hand, place them on your chin, and bring your chin to your chest. Hold it there and breathe. Release your head, and repeat with your left hand.

YOGA ASANAS AND PRANAYAMA EXERCISES TO HEAL THE FIFTH CHAKRA

Try these exercises to help heal and align the Vishuddha chakra.

To view a video demo of these exercises, go to
www.youtube.com/c/MichelleFondinAuthor.
Click on the Playlists tab, and select
Chakra Healing Asanas & Pranayamas.
Scroll down the list until you find the one you're looking for.

Ujjayi **Breath:** Often referred to as the ocean breath or affectionately coined the Darth Vader breath, the ujjayi breath is excellent for toning the throat and calming nerves. This breath brings heat to the body and therefore is yang in nature. To begin the ujjayi breath, sit tall and close your eyes. Pretend you're going to fog up a pair of glasses to clean them, and exhale the word *ha*. Now close your lips and exhale the same way but with your mouth closed. Inhale and exhale the word *ha*. This results in a partial constriction of your throat. You are breathing from the lower belly, inflating the belly as you inhale and contracting it as you exhale. In the beginning, it's difficult to inhale the word *ha*, but with practice it becomes easier. Once you get the hang of it, see if you can prolong each inhalation and exhalation to the count of four. Use this breathing technique anytime you're feeling stressed.

Lion's Breath — *Simhasana*: This silly-looking breath is effective at toning the throat, mouth, and jaw, and clearing out the lungs and bronchial passages. To practice the lion's breath, sit on your heels with your knees wide open and place your hands on the floor in front of you. If it's challenging to sit this way, you can stand and place your feet wide apart instead. Take in a deep breath through your nose, and as you exhale, open your mouth wide, stick out your tongue, and say the word *ha* emphasizing the *h* on the exhale, as if you are a lion roaring. If you want to add another physical component to complete the asana, bring up your hands and make claws as you exhale. It's great for releasing negative energy.

Bridge Pose — *Setu Bandhasana*: Begin by lying on your back with your knees bent and your feet flat on the floor. Place your feet hip-width apart and parallel, your toes forward, and your arms alongside you with your palms facing down. Press your palms down and lift your pelvis up. If you can, bring your hands together on the mat underneath your pelvis and interlace your fingers. Walk your shoulders inward toward your spine, and lift your pelvis even higher. Look straight at the ceiling, and keep your head steady. Hold for five to ten breaths. To lower, separate your hands, bring your palms to the floor, and lower your pelvis to the ground. As a counterpose, bring both knees to your chest and roll gently side to side to massage your back. Bridge pose stimulates the thyroid, parathyroid, and thymus glands.

Shoulderstand — *Salamba Sarvangasana*: Shoulderstand is a more advanced pose, so if you're a beginner, do it at a wall (see below for instructions) or with a spotter. Place a thinly folded blanket or towel on your mat, and lie down so that the blanket is underneath your head, neck, and shoulders. Bring your arms alongside you with your palms facing down. Bend your knees with your feet flat on the floor. Press your hands to the floor, and bring your legs straight into the air while lifting your lower back. Bring your hands up to support your back, and move your elbows inward toward your spine. Keep your head straight and steady; do not turn it to the side. If you would prefer to use a wall, start in the same position with your mat perpendicular to the wall. Bend your knees and place your feet against the wall. Press your feet into the wall to lift your pelvis, support your lower back with your hands, and walk your feet up the wall. If you feel stable, bring one foot away from the wall and then the other to extend the legs straight up toward the ceiling. Remain in the pose for a few breaths or a few minutes depending on your ability level. To lower, bring your bent knees toward your forehead and gently roll your back to the floor. If continuing with the sequence shown here, move on to plow pose. If you're ready to wind down, do fish pose (*matsyasana*; see page 174) or reclining butterfly pose (see page 55).

Plow Pose — *Halasana*: To begin, lie down with a thinly folded blanket underneath your head and neck. Rest your arms alongside your torso with your palms facing down. Bend both knees with your feet flat on the floor. Press into your hands and lift your legs. With your legs joined and straight, bring them over your head until your toes touch the floor above your head. You will be folding your body completely in half. You can either leave your arms on the floor or bend your elbows and support your back with your hands. Hold the pose for several breaths. To come out of the pose, lower your knees toward your forehead and gently lower your back to the floor, one vertebrae at a time. To recover, do reclining butterfly pose (see page 55) or hug your knees to your chest, and roll your back out side to side.

 Healing the Emotional and Energetic Body

For many of us, one of the hardest things to do is to speak truth. I'm not referring to telling the truth, which at times is challenging in and of itself. I'm talking about speaking your inner truth, the truth that resides within your heart. The truth that is the pure essence within your personal soul, the voice that comes from your highest Self and gives authenticity to your words. It speaks of who you are as an individual and brings light to your uniqueness in every way.

In the third and fourth chakras, your personality develops to formulate your passions and love. But it's in the fifth chakra that these formulations are exposed to the world through your words and verbal expression.

Fear of rejection or of not fitting in may be a reason why you feel you can't share who you are. Yet who you are is what God breathed into your soul, and you will feel balanced only when you share that with the world.

Living in Truth

Far from being an easy task for most of us, living in truth means living authentically in every moment. When you take this to heart and put it into practice, you truly realize how incredibly challenging it is. It is humbling and ego-crushing, in a way. Unless you are consciously working at this, you aren't generally cognizant of how much untruth can infiltrate your life. Most of the untruths aren't harmful or pivotal to changing your destiny, but they are like little grains of sand that can build up to a mountain.

Think of the reasons why you might not tell the truth or the entire truth. Sometimes we don't say the truth because it's not convenient, such as telling your boss that you were late because you were stuck in traffic rather than because you got into an argument with your spouse. Or maybe the untruth comes from fear of embarrassment. For example, you accidentally schedule a date with a new hot guy on the same night as you had already committed to another date with another guy who isn't so hot. So you lie and say you're sick. Or perhaps you tell an untruth because you fear rejection or you feel bad for the other person. There are many reasons why you might tell an untruth, and most of them are linked to fear. Fear is a low and slow energy. Once you reach the fifth chakra your body, mind, and soul are already vibrating at a higher frequency so you can easily connect to your spiritual self. Any untruth or lie you tell inside or out will corrode the link between you and your higher self. Therefore it's not about the bent reality that you're telling but rather your alignment with your own integrity and the higher vibrations of truth and love.

BEING AUTHENTIC VERSUS BEING NICE

Authenticity is about lifting the false masks of your identity as a person and revealing who you are to the world. We all wear masks. Sometimes we wear the mask of someone who works, who plays, who is a spouse, friend, son, daughter, sister, brother, and so on. And we tend to wear different masks for different people. Living in the truth is about discarding all those masks and instead exposing yourself to the world as you are. People who live authentically show little difference in their attitudes and appearances no matter who is before them. Sometimes these people are referred to as "genuine and real" or even "down-to-earth."

If, on the other hand, you are constantly worried about pleasing others or afraid of what others might think of you, you are not only wearing masks but also changing those masks depending on who is in front of you. Being nice, or people pleasing, is the antithesis of truth. It's impossible to be genuine or authentic and be a people pleaser. If you morph into what other people want or what you think they want, you deny who you are and your needs and desires.

You can begin to counter this tendency by first finding out what you truly want, need, and desire. Get to know yourself and your true nature. For example, if you hate golf but you go golfing with the guys every weekend because you want to fit in or to climb the corporate ladder, you aren't being true to yourself by doing it. Eventually your dislike for golfing will show through and the guys will figure out you're just doing it to get ahead. Your actions will backfire in a way that will be disadvantageous to you.

When I was a young stay-at-home mom, I noticed that all the other moms around me spent most of their time volunteering at the elementary school and carting their kids around to several sporting teams and other extracurricular activities. I fell into the trap of wanting to be like them. I thought I should be the perfect mom and that I could achieve that by doing the things they did. I exhausted myself by volunteering my time and chauffeuring my kids to many activities. Then one day I woke up and found myself miserable. I also noticed that my kids were miserable too. All the volunteering took time away from parenting. And the overscheduling didn't give my kids time to play and be kids. Once I realized this, I cut volunteering down to once a month and made my kids choose at most one extracurricular activity at a time. Everyone was happier when I was truthful to myself.

REFLECTING ON SPEAKING TRUTH

Try this interesting exercise. During the day, focus on your words and see if they match how you truly feel. Resist the temptation to judge or admonish yourself; just notice. You may be amazed to discover times when you don't think you're "stretching the truth" but you are. Keep in mind that I'm not talking about joking around or exaggerating to prove a point but rather deliberately changing the truth to mislead another person or yourself in any way. For example, if you get on the scale to weigh yourself and you weigh 160 pounds, but you tell your spouse, who asks, that the scale read 150 pounds, that's deliberate. You might think, "Well, what's the harm in that? It's just a number on a scale." That might be so, but if it weren't a big deal, why would you change the number?

Ultimately, speaking truth and being mindful of your inner truth is about flexing a muscle so you can live a life of excellence, marked by coherence between body, mind, and spirit. The more you flex your muscles of deception, the bigger they get. And the more you flex your truthfulness muscles, the bigger those get. In the end, you have greater gains when your truthfulness muscles are flexed and toned.

Living in and speaking truth doesn't mean you always have to tell all. It is your absolute right to say things such as "I'd rather not say," "I'm not sure right now," or even "Now isn't the right time for me to express this." If truth means you will hurt someone and that isn't where you'd like to go with the conversation, you can always stay silent, unless staying silent means you might harm them. For example, if your friend asks you if you love her new red dress and you don't like it at all, you could either stay silent or say something like, "I really like the flowered dress you wore last week." You're using a softener to avoid hurting her feelings, but you're not lying. However, if she says to you, "What do you think about this new guy I'm dating?" And you google the guy and find out he has a police record and you don't tell her, then you could potentially be harming her by not revealing the truth. Do you see the difference?

As you go through your day with this exercise, say to yourself, "Is what I'm about to say going to hurt my integrity in any way?" and "Will I be disconnecting from my spiritual self by saying what I'm about to say?" You'll notice that if you can answer those questions honestly, you'll go about your day honoring truthfulness.

Healing the Spiritual Body

Gaining the awareness of the fifth chakra is like awakening from a deep slumber. You begin to see things differently. Words spoken or written take on new meaning. As you emerge from the darkness of the lower chakras, spiritual truths seem to fall into place and link together like the pieces of a puzzle that seemed so complicated before. You may find yourself on a sudden spiritual journey, seeking to take in as much information as you possibly can. It's an exciting time for you as you begin to wonder where all this wonderful truth has been hiding your whole life.

Awakening to the Truth

Have you ever read a really good book with an important message and then picked it back up several years later and gotten a completely different message? That is what it feels like to awaken to spiritual truths. An old adage says, "When the student is ready, the teacher will appear." At this stage of our chakra journey, we have traveled far into a spiritual plane where things just start to make sense.

You might feel that before this moment, you were like a piece of seaweed being tossed around by the waves with absolutely no control over your thoughts, feelings, emotions, and destiny. Now you're beginning to understand that you *are* the ocean. How empowering it is to realize that when you align yourself with the creative force of the entire universe, everything is possible.

You are at the point in your spiritual development that you are so ecstatic you want to shout from the rooftops to everyone around you, "Don't you see this? Don't you understand? This is amazing!" But alas, everyone around you is not on your spiritual path, and they don't understand. They are like you were before you awakened. In the beginning, it can be frustrating. You want to share all this wonderful knowledge. You want others to see that we are not our bodies but spiritual beings having a human experience. With the knowledge gained from your heart chakra, you can reach back in and have compassion for those who have not yet seen what you see.

Your faith grows by leaps and bounds as you test out this new spiritual awareness. You may be shy to share your joy, but it's necessary that you do so in order to share these spiritual truths with others, just as they were shared with you.

VISHUDDHA GUIDED MEDITATION

Sit comfortably and close your eyes. Bring your attention and awareness to the area of your throat. If it's chilly in the room, cover your throat with a warm scarf. Or if you prefer, you can use your hands: crisscross your hands to make the shape of a butterfly, and gently place your palms against your throat. This will bring warmth and healing energy to the fifth chakra. Set the intention to bring healing to your neck, throat, thyroid gland, parathyroid glands, jaw, mouth, tongue, vocal cords, and ears. As you settle in to relaxing all these parts of your body, ask the question, "How do I know my inner truth?" By simply asking the question, you'll find that the answers will appear. Then bring your awareness back to the word *truth*. Ask your higher self to access your inner truth.

Bring to your awareness different aspects of your

life, and continue to ask your higher self, "What is my inner truth here?" Start with the most important things in your life, such as your family, friends, and other relationships, then go to your personal health and well-being, continually asking yourself, "What is my inner truth here?" Next, expand outward to your work or career, and ask yourself, "What is my inner truth here?" Then go to your passions, gifts, and talents: "What is my inner truth here?" Next, consider the material items in your life — finances, money, home, cars, and other material goods — and ask yourself, "What is my inner truth here?" Finally, go to your spirituality, your beliefs, your ideals, your values, and ask, "What is my inner truth here?" Take some time to go over other areas of your life that come up for you now, repeating the same question: "What is my inner truth here?"

Listen to what comes up. Acknowledge it with a nod. Try not to judge whatever comes to you in this conversation with your higher self. When you're finished, thank your higher self for all the insight. You can seal the meditation by chanting the mantra sound *HUM* three times.

When you feel ready, you can slowly open your eyes and return to activity. Since this guided meditation has brought you some revelations, you may want to write down what came to you during the meditation.

ENERGY-BODY HEALING WITH GEMS AND COLORS

The color sky blue is associated with the fifth chakra.

Lapis lazuli, known as the "stone of truth," is great for speaking your truth. You can also use aquamarine and turquoise.

You can wear or hold to your throat chakra the stones blue kyanite and blue iolite to help enhance clairaudient or psychic hearing abilities.

Fifth Chakra Mindfulness Ideas to Ponder

1. When I communicate with others, I will keep in mind that it's not the words that create beautiful stories, but the spaces between the words. And it's not the musical notes that create melodious music, but the pauses between the notes. I'm creating space in my communication. I'm pausing, listening fully, and allowing the space to create beautiful conversations.
2. Revealing my inner truth is the only way to authenticity.
3. Honesty is the way I express my self-love and my integrity.
4. I remain open to all forms of communication, and I honor others' needs to express themselves in many ways.
5. As I live more in truth, more truth will be revealed to me.

6

THE THIRD-EYE CHAKRA
Ajna

ELEMENT: Light
COLOR: Indigo
MANTRA SOUND: *SHAM*

The sixth chakra is a special place on our chakra journey. Anatomically, we have arrived at the area of the third eye, which is located between the two eyebrows and the two physical eyes. The sixth chakra includes the eyes and the pineal gland. Ajna is our center of intuition and clairvoyance, or seeing things beyond the physical.

Relatively speaking, the descriptions of the first five chakras have been fairly grounded and hopefully relatable to your daily life. Please bear with me throughout the description of the sixth chakra, as it will be more esoteric.

The world we live in is made up of opposites. Where there is up, there is down. Where there is day, there is night. Where there is darkness, there is light. No matter how hard we try to only have half of something, its opposite always tends to show up somehow. As happy as you can be one day, you know in the back of your mind that something can happen to make you sad. But the upside is, when you're sad, you can be fairly certain that it won't last and that you will eventually experience happiness again, if you're patient. This principle of opposites is called duality.

When you were born, you came into this world of duality. You began life on earth, and shortly thereafter you realized that you will die someday.

According to Tantra yoga philosophy, we can transcend this world of duality while we're still living. We don't have to experience death to appreciate our state of perfection wherein suffering no longer exists. We can have this experience while we're alive.

In the first five chakras we're stuck with the experience of our five senses, the *tanmantras*; with the five elements, the mahabhutas; and with the three gunas, or states of being. The first five chakras are also bound to the three doshas as well as the alternating energies of yin and yang, which are representative of the Ida and Pingala nadis. As you can see, up until this point, we were bound to the ebb and flow of many factors that influenced the experiences of our existence.

Not anymore. Once you reach the Ajna chakra, you're able to go beyond all these factors. The Ida and Pingala nadis end in the nostrils. For the sixth chakra, the two physical eyes represent the Ida and Pingala nadis, and the third eye represents the Shushumna nadi. Remember that the Shushumna nadi is the central nadi that runs through the spinal cord connecting all seven main chakras. The physical eyes see the past and present, and the third eye sees the future. Lastly, the physical eyes represent the sun and moon, and the third eye represents fire or intense light.

This beautiful quote by Dr. K. O. Paulose portrays the essence of the sixth chakra: "Ajna is where time ceases to exist.

There is no past, no present and no future. Ajna will help you break down the barriers between your individual self and teach you to blend with the cosmic mind in single-pointed consciousness. This is the chakra wherein duality ends. There is no light and dark; no good and evil. Unconditional truth is the essence of Ajna."

The color we attribute to the third-eye chakra is indigo. The mantra, or bija (seed) sound, we vocalize for the sixth chakra is *SHAM*.

Sixth Chakra Ailments

Ailments of the Ajna chakra include blindness, eyestrain, blurred vision, headaches, hallucinations, difficulty concentrating, and nightmares. Memory problems can also be a sixth chakra disorder.

Sixth Chakra Energy

If you have never experienced a transcendent state, Ajna's energy may be difficult to understand. You might even have a hard time believing that something like this exists. Let me give you an example to help you recognize that you have already experienced the transcendent quality of the sixth chakra.

Have you ever experienced your sense of intuition through a hunch or inner knowing? Have you had a clear sense about a person or situation but no idea how you knew it? Let's say you're in the market to buy a new car. You shop around and find a particular vehicle that you would like to buy. The car salesman shows you the top-of-the-line model with all the bells and whistles. You explain you want the basic model with heated front seats but nothing else extra. He convinces you that he can get you a great deal, fantastic trade-in value, and perfect financing on the car he showed you. Reluctantly you agree to let him write up the paperwork. Three hours later he says he's crunched all the numbers and presents you with a bill that is $5,000 more than you wanted to spend. Defeated, you're about to sign on the dotted line when something inside you says, "Stop!" You put down your pen and tell the salesman, "I think I need to shop around some more. I think I can get a better deal elsewhere." He tries to convince you that you could never in a million years find a better deal on such a car. Listening to your intuition, you leave and head off to another dealership where you're able to buy the same top-of-the-line model for $5,000 less, exactly what you wanted to pay in the first place and with more amenities. That is transcendence.

You might argue that your decision to leave the first dealership was pure logic since you know through life experience when you're being taken to the cleaners. But your hunch wasn't based on factual information, not unless you had called every single car dealership in your area with the specs on that same car and had already gathered the information before declining the first deal. It came from an inner knowing, a small voice that told you to get out while you still could.

If you've ever experienced telepathy or meaningful coincidence, you've also tapped into your sixth chakra. Have you ever thought about someone you hadn't seen or spoken to in a long time, and the mere experience of thinking about her caused her to call you out of the blue? Or maybe you thought about a book you really wanted to read, and a friend walked up to you and said, "I was out shopping, saw this book, and thought of you. Would you like to have it?" That happened to me while I was living in France. I was helping my father-in-law, who was having some health issues. I was thinking about a book I had read several years before, *8 Weeks to Optimum Health* by

Dr. Andrew Weil. I knew that if I could give it to him, it might change his life. But I didn't know where to find it or if it was even translated into French. That day I went to the supermarket and walked past a bargain bin full of books. I glanced down and there was *8 Weeks to Optimum Health* in French and on sale. It was crazy. That is what happens when you access your sixth chakra fully.

Many people brush off events like that as mere coincidence or happenstance. My answer to them is, "Really?" What are the chances that a book, originally published in 1997, would find itself in a bargain bin in a grocery store in France in 2006, among all the hundreds of thousands of books that exist, and at the exact same time that I was at that grocery store? I would bet that the probability is close to zero. That event was divinely orchestrated as a result of my meditating and living in a higher state of consciousness.

Meaningful coincidences or synchronistic events begin to occur when you align yourself with the spiritual energy that resides in the Ajna chakra. Life becomes easier and more fulfilling. You experience more joy, and your life becomes more meaningful.

Our Societal Relationship with the Sixth Chakra

We have not yet reached a point in our society where sixth chakra consciousness exists for the majority. If that were the case, there would be no such thing as good people and bad people, therefore no wars would formulate. There would be no push-pull of the ego, and thus we wouldn't be concerned with competition or getting ahead of other people. A mind-set of abundance would reign everywhere as we would realize that there is enough on this planet for everyone. Crime would be nonexistent as a result of wealth consciousness. If everything was light, then there would be no darkness.

The feeling of interconnectedness would end the debate as to whether or not we need to take care of our planet. The answer would be obvious. Daily life would flow in greater peace and harmony.

The emergence of spiritual enlightenment is in its infancy in the West. There is certainly more awareness than in the past one hundred years, but greater darkness as well. We have shifted from world wars to wars on ourselves and our health. Illness in society as a whole reflects the state of consciousness of its people. According to the Centers for Disease Control and Prevention, half of all US adults, or 133 million people, suffer from at least one chronic disease. Disease cannot exist in sixth chakra consciousness. By synchronizing with mind, body, spirit, and the entire universe, you are vibrating at such a fast speed that the lower energies of disease cannot take hold in you.

Let me give you an example. Perhaps there has been a time in your life when you were living in bliss. Your career was great. You were deeply in love. Your family life was balanced, and you woke up every morning feeling fantastic. You felt on top of the world. Maybe that time lasted for a week, a month, or a year. But do you remember that during that time, when you felt like you could take on the world, you didn't get sick? People around you were getting colds or the flu, but not you. You were untouched by disease even though you were exposed to it. Inversely, perhaps there was a time when everything was going wrong. You lost your job, your car broke down, and your dog died all in one week. You were stressed, sad, and worried, and on top of it all you got hit with a killer bronchial infection.

I would suggest that if you want to live a life that is disease-free, along with following the other principles offered in this book, stay away from disease consciousness. Turn off the TV or radio when prescription drug ads come on, and even try to avoid advertisements for hospitals, cancer treatment centers, and other medical centers. You don't want any of that energy anywhere near you. It will lower your vibrational frequency. If friends or family talk about the flu epidemic or the Zika virus, ask them to please change the subject. If you feel a minor ache or pain, try not to surf the internet looking for diseases. Instead, do some yoga breathing, meditate, or change your diet. I know people who feel a small pain, and after browsing disease possibilities, they're off to their doctor with a self-diagnosis. Other than getting yearly checkups, wouldn't it be better to not have to rely on doctors so much? Your body is a healing machine. Consider it as such.

Wouldn't it be wonderful if instead of medical advertisements, we had motivational advertisements? Imagine where your thoughts would go if you saw a big billboard that read "Your body is a healing machine. You're healthy now," then you opened your internet browser and a pop-up ad read "You have extraordinary energy!" Most medical companies would go out of business.

When we let go of the belief that disease is a given, we can then evolve in consciousness as a society.

Living Life in the Ajna Chakra

The person who dwells in the Ajna chakra lives a magical but disciplined life. The gifts that come with sixth chakra consciousness only come with the greatest amount of austerity and adherence to steadfast principles. It's no wonder that only a select few ever attain this level of consciousness. The work required to gain these gifts is a tough and often lonely road.

Others around you may not understand why you need to meditate for an hour a day or practice yoga daily. They may not get why you buy only organic food, recycle, or consistently give to charities. They might tease you for never drinking alcohol, using drugs, or taking any substances that will harm your body. They may find you weak for never arguing with others or trying to prove that you're right. And they certainly won't understand why you prefer silence to blaring music or a loud television.

By living in the Ajna chakra you give up a great many things, but you gain much more in return. You live in bliss and joy every day of your life. The resources you need seem to appear out of nowhere. You begin to see into the future and know the places and people to avoid. Your life unfolds effortlessly and easily. Many people living in this state have the power to heal. And when you are in the presence of others, they feel at peace.

Recognizing Sixth Chakra Imbalances

Practicing meditation and living a life of austerity are not the only ways to obtain the level of transcendence most people seek. Beware of fast tracks to transcendence. Some people will try to obtain sixth chakra transcendence by destructive means such as extreme fasting, drugs, alcohol, and other types of addictive behavior. You can have momentary journeys into bliss by flooding your brain with addictive substances or by depriving the brain of oxygen, food, or water. But these things always come with a price. By forcing yourself into higher states of consciousness, you create a karmic debt that must be repaid. Often the lows include plummeting back into the most primal and basic areas of the first chakra, where you're surrounded by fear, shame, and guilt. Since all of us are seeking a greater spiritual connection on some level, it can be tempting to try to take a shortcut to transcendent bliss. However, anything worth having is also worth working toward.

Accepting Sixth Chakra Gifts

If you're not already living in the sixth chakra state of consciousness at least some of the time, it can be scary to accept the gifts of this chakra. You may be reluctant to follow your intuition or trust your visions, whether they come from within or as outer visual experiences.

Accepting sixth chakra gifts can give you an edge over others who don't accept them. Your power of intuition can save you a lot of pain and heartache. It can help you make better choices and guide you along your life path with greater ease. The power of dreaming and visualization can get you to your desires and life purpose at lightning speed. The sixth chakra transcends time and space. In the universal realm, manifestation is not linear. It does not await the perfect time and place. You can take quantum leaps in progress through the power of visualization, daydreaming, and following your intuition.

I met this woman at a meeting of Al-Anon, a recovery group for people who are affected by someone else's drinking. She was a nice person with a big heart. She shared with me that she had been in the program for over forty-nine years. She said she was still working on the issues that plagued her from the beginning. Many other women in the program seemed to be experiencing the same. They had spent years and often decades in the program, going over the mistakes of the past and often repeating the same mistakes in the present. I often hear this story of people who stay in therapy for many years. I don't believe in getting stuck in this sort of holding pattern. For true spiritual development to occur, you must continually grow. Programs and self-help books are wonderful and great. There are layers to personal growth that can and do unfold with repetition. However, if you find yourself repeating the same destructive behavior or mulling over past behavior, feelings, or emotions, you will find it difficult to reach the sixth chakra level of consciousness. Instead of daydreaming about how you have this defect or that ingrained behavior or emotion, visualize yourself as healed and strong. Spend time daydreaming about living in a different mind-set and staying there. Living your life differently is as easy as a decision. My philosophy: get the lesson and move on.

We all have a limited amount of time on this planet. You might have seventy, eighty, ninety, or one hundred years total. With the knowledge that your time is limited, why not make the best use of it by working *with* universal energy instead of against it? When you make the decision to accept this spiritual aspect of who you are, you will see yourself grow by leaps and bounds.

Healing Ajna

DAILY AFFIRMATION
I follow the path of truth.

 Healing the Physical Body

To help relieve blockages or imbalances in the sixth chakra, it's important to choose life-affirming foods, clean water, and a healthy, toxin-free living environment. Move your body daily and practice meditation. Living in this manner is essential as you awaken each of the chakras. However, if you wish to experience the physical lightness that brings to you the gifts of the sixth chakra, you must keep your body free of toxins. Of course, you can't control everything in your environment, but try to control what you can.

You will have increased ability to access your intuition if you spend time in nature. Your body will sync up with the rhythms of nature, and you will experience more flow in your life.

YOGA EYE EXERCISES

Great for strengthening the cones and rods in the eyes as well as stimulating the brain, these yoga eye exercises take only two to three minutes to do. Remove your glasses or contact lenses. Sit tall with your palms on your lap facing up. Keep your head steady. Repeat each of the following three exercises ten times:

Look up to the right and down to the left. Then look up to the left and down to the right.

Look side to side, as if you were trying to look at each ear.

Look up between your eyebrows, and look down toward your chin.

Finally, look toward your nose, and hold for twenty to thirty seconds. When you're finished, rub your hands together to create friction and heat. Place the heels of your hands over your eyes, and hold for about thirty seconds. Still holding your hands over your eyes, gently move the heels of your hands in a circular motion over your eyes to massage them. When you're finished, remove your hands and open your eyes.

LIGHT THERAPY

In addition to eye exercises, you can strengthen your sense of sight and help heal a whole host of diseases by using light therapy. The best source of light therapy, of course, is the sun. Never stare directly at the sun. However, you can stare at the sun with your eyes closed. You can also try circular eye motions: with your eyes closed, look toward the sun and trace its shape by moving your eyes in a clockwise motion and then switching to counterclockwise. Do this sunning therapy for ten minutes daily. In the winter you can achieve a similar effect by using a full-spectrum light box designed for light therapy. According to a Mayo Clinic article, the light box should provide an exposure to 10,000 lux of light and emit as little ultraviolet light as possible to avoid skin and eye damage. In the same way that you wouldn't look directly at the sun for your eye exercises, avoid staring directly at the light box. Consult your eye doctor before using any type of light therapy for your eyes if you have glaucoma, cataracts, or eye damage from diabetes.

YOGA ASANAS AND PRANAYAMA EXERCISES TO HEAL THE SIXTH CHAKRA

Practice these breathing techniques and poses to help balance the Ajna chakra.

To view a video demo of these exercises, go to
www.youtube.com/c/MichelleFondinAuthor.
Click on the Playlists tab, and select
Chakra Healing Asanas & Pranayamas.
Scroll down the list until you find the one you're looking for.

Alternate-Nostril Breathing — *Nadi Shodhana*: The practice of nadi shodhana synchronizes the hemispheres of the brain. Begin by sitting with your back straight and your eyes closed. Place your left hand on your lap, with your palm facing up. Take your right hand and place your index and middle fingers on the third eye in between your eyebrows. Gently rest your right thumb on your right nostril. Rest the inside of your folded ring finger on your left nostril. To begin, inhale through both nostrils and exhale through both nostrils with your lips closed. Block your right nostril with your thumb, and inhale through your left nostril for the count of two. Block both nostrils and hold for six. Then exhale through your right nostril for the count of four. Inhale through your right nostril for two, hold both for six, and then exhale through your left nostril for four. Keep the same counts as you alternate. Repeat this breathing pattern for two to five minutes.

Bee Breath — *Bhramari*: This breathing technique helps clear sinuses, alleviate headaches, and calm nerves. Sit in a comfortable position with your spine tall, and close your eyes. Gently press the middle and ring finger of each hand against your eyes, covering them completely. Press your thumbs into your inner ears to close off your hearing. Rest your pinkies on your upper cheeks and your index fingers slightly above your eyebrows. Take a deep breath through your nose and into your belly, and exhale by saying *HUM* or *OM*, emphasizing the *mmmmm* sound and prolonging it for the entire exhalation. You will feel the vibration throughout your head. Repeat for at least ten breaths. You will feel invigorated after completing the bee breath.

Eagle Pose — *Garudasana*: Eagle pose is great for cultivating focus and one-pointed attention. Begin by standing on your mat with your feet parallel. Bend your knees and lift your right leg up to cross it over your left. If you can, wrap your toes behind your left calf. You will now be in a seated-chair squat with one leg wrapped around the other. If it's too difficult to wrap your toes, place your right foot on the side of your left leg. You can also place a yoga block next to your left foot and place your right toes on the block. Next, bring your arms up and bend them so they look like goalposts. Wrap your right arm underneath your left, and thread it around until your two hands meet at the top. Your arms will be interlaced together like your legs. With your arms wrapped, bring both palms together. Your focal point will be your hands. Bring your elbows up and your shoulders down. Hold the pose for four to six breaths, and then repeat on the other side.

Dolphin Pose — *Ardha Pincha Mayurasana*: Dolphin pose is a mild inversion, or a yoga pose in which the head is at a lower position than the heart. As a general rule, inversions are good for all the upper chakras. Even though dolphin pose looks easy, it's actually quite challenging as it requires some upper body strength. You can work your way up to holding dolphin pose by taking frequent breaks. Dolphin pose is also good practice to build your strength for a yoga headstand.

Begin on your hands and knees on your mat. Lay your forearms on the mat with your elbows directly underneath your shoulders. Fold your hands together in front of you, and lock your shoulders back to create a stable base. Your hands and elbows will form a triangle. Gently lift your knees off the floor and walk your feet toward your elbows until you're in an upside-down letter *V*. Your head will float above the floor. Lift your tailbone high into the sky. To enhance the energy toward the Ajna chakra, lift your head so the third eye is facing directly down toward the earth. Stay in the pose for four to six breaths, then lower your knees to the floor and take a child's pose as a counterpose: lower your hips to the floor, and then extend your torso forward and rest it between your thighs, with your forehead on the floor.

 ## Healing the Emotional and Energetic Body

Then God said, "Let there be light," and there was light.
And God saw that the light was good.
Then he separated light from the darkness.
— GENESIS 1:3–4

A great obstacle in healing the emotional body, especially at the sixth chakra level of consciousness, is the struggle of light versus dark. Earnest spiritual seekers can be so interested in attainment of enlightenment that they forget some crucial steps along the path.

In the beginning of the chapter I discussed the duality dynamic of this world. The push-pull of the world of opposites doesn't only live in your environment; it also lives in you. There are aspects within you that seem to work against everything you stand for on your spiritual path. Yet there they are, either ever present or looming around the corner. The novice on the spiritual path will try to push them away, hoping that they will never return. But these shadows must be confronted and accepted in order to experience the light fully. A perfect example is if you never saw darkness, you could never experience the night sky filled with stars, planets, and other astral bodies.

Often it is through your own darkness that you discover the light. In the Bible, God created light out of the darkness since the darkness came first. My experience with cancer enabled me to help countless people through my writing about healing. When I talk to people in recovery from alcohol and drug addiction, they all say that they would never have arrived at the spiritual lives they now live if it weren't for the dark days of addiction.

We have all seen instances in the media demonstrating that pushing away the darkness only makes things worse. Look at the sex scandals of politicians, stories of embezzlement, and improper use of campaign funds.

One of the greatest teachers I ever had, Dr. David Simon, used to say, "You can do all the meditation in the world, but if you don't work on emotional healing, you can't reach enlightenment." Emotional healing doesn't mean you have to spend twenty years in therapy. It simply means facing your demons, the shadow aspects of you that aren't fun to look at. Invite them in and have a conversation with them. Tell them they aren't going to rule your life anymore.

I used to have quite an issue with anxiety. At different periods in my life, it ruined my daily experiences. I became paralyzed by stories in my head that, for the most part, simply weren't true. But I let my mind entertain those stories. I used to say in jest that the great thing about being a writer is that I have a wild imagination, and the worst thing about being a writer is that I have a wild imagination. Learning and practicing meditation saved me because I learned that I can control my thoughts and their direction.

The best way to face your shadows is to transmute them. Transform the shadow energy into something great that can help humanity. Send light into the darkness. For example, if your shadow is that you succumb to obsessive cleaning and organizing in your home, you could start a business where you help others organize closets and living spaces. If you're a shopaholic, you can contact your local women's shelter and ask them what they need in a care box. You can then use your shopping skills to find the best prices to make care boxes for women and children in a safe home. The greatest thing about being human is that you are human. There is no reason to be ashamed of your weaknesses or your shadows as long as you are not harming anyone, including yourself. In fact, it's often when we bring our shadows into the light that their power dissipates. Professional help can assist you in this process, but sometimes a simple decision to act is all you need.

 ## Healing the Spiritual Body

Meditation is the primary practice that will help you attain the sixth chakra level of awareness. Talk about meditation is bubbling under the surface of American culture these days, and efforts to include meditation in daily activities are popping up in hospitals, corporations, and even schools. More than the word *meditation*, you may hear the word *mindfulness*, which refers to a type of meditation. As a meditation teacher, I find the word *mindfulness* to be a bit of a misnomer when it comes to the ultimate goal of meditation. Awareness is certainly the key to everything we have discussed up until now. You must be aware of your thoughts, words, and actions, as well as your body and mind. However, when I think of mindfulness, I think of concentration or fullness of the mind. To meditate, you need focus instead of concentration, and release of the mind rather than fullness of it.

Most people come to meditation saying, "I'm too much in

my mind! Get me out of it!" You are literally going out of your mind in meditation. (That pun was completely intended.) Everyone has experienced the effects of monkey mind. Your mind flits from thought to thought like a monkey swinging from branch to branch. Without awareness that you are the thinker of your thoughts, you become subject to the mind's unwieldy habit of flitting about with no sense of control. It comes as no surprise that millions of people suffer from anxiety and depression. If you are under the impression that you have no control over your thoughts and the strong impulses of the mind, of course you have reason to feel anxious. However, the good news is that you do have control. You simply need to learn tools to exercise the control muscle.

By realizing that there are separate roles at play inside you, you can harness the forces of your mind and get it to do what you want. You achieve this by cajoling your mind rather than forcing it to go in the direction you desire. How do most of us try to control the mind? Let's suppose you're trying to break a bad habit, such as eating a chocolate bar every night. You may try to break this habit by setting a goal such as not eating chocolate at all or eating chocolate only once per week. Then you might try to abstain from chocolate by not purchasing it, distracting yourself in other ways, or replacing it with something else. All these ways can and do work. But they all involve forcing the mind into distraction. If you have ever tried doing something like this, you know that it's difficult and tiring. You really have to fight the mind frequently. Your mind will tell you things such as "Chocolate isn't that bad. Studies have shown it has antioxidants that make you healthy" or "You've had a rough day today; don't you deserve a little chocolate?" And on and on goes the mind with great arguments to separate you

from your goal. The thing about fighting or using strong re-
solve to get to where you want to go is that it's fatiguing rather
than empowering. Eventually you will get tired of the battle
and give up.

Now let's compare the above method with cajoling the mind
by going out of your mind. When you meditate, you are not in
your mind. You are accessing your spirit or the part of you that
was never born and therefore can never die. Your spirit is the
part of you that is eternal. My guru Dr. Wayne W. Dyer used to
say that when you talk to yourself, there are two people: you and
your Self. The Self with a capital *S* is the higher self I'm speaking of. The other self, known as the ego, is the one who tries to
push through toward your goals and leaves you tired. The higher
self is the part of you who only wants good and can harness
the power of intuition. When you get out of your mind through
meditation, you gain greater access to your higher self.

One common misconception about meditation is that
you're stopping all the activities of the mind. The job of the
mind is to think thoughts. It will always do that, no matter what. Through meditation you can lower the number of
thoughts and evolve your thoughts to get you closer to what
you desire, but you will not stop all thought. As you get out of
your mind, also referred to as transcendence, you strengthen
your relationship with your spirit or higher self. Then you return back to the mind with love and acceptance. With these
higher qualities of spirit, you cajole the mind into thinking
thoughts that lovingly, effortlessly, and easily help you.

The chaos of the monkey mind subsides, and you are left
with a mind that thinks more clearly. The more you meditate,
the clearer your mind can think and the more in touch you
become with your intuition.

AJNA GUIDED MEDITATION

Sit or lie comfortably and close your eyes. Place your awareness on the area between your eyebrows at the third eye. If you want to make your awareness clearer, lick your thumb, and then press the moisture on the third eye. Take in a couple of deep belly breaths, exhaling completely. With your focus still on the third eye, ask your higher self to step forward. Your higher self, also referred to as the witness, is the one who has always been there. It is the still, small voice inside you that always gives you truth. It is the aspect of you that was there before you were born and that will be with you after you die. Your higher self is ever present, ever witnessing, and always acts according to your higher good. Greet your higher self and welcome it in.

You are going on a journey with your higher self from the time of your earliest memory. Think back to your first memory. What was it? Who was there? What did the scenery look like? What were you wearing? What were others wearing? Do you remember your witnessing presence being there? What wisdom did it share with you then?

Next, go to a memory in your early childhood years, between the ages of six and twelve. Is there a particular moment that sticks out for you? Do you remember your higher self being there and letting you know what you should do? Did you follow your inner witness, or did you go against it?

Next, fast-forward to your teenage years between the ages of thirteen and nineteen. What moment comes to mind during these years? Who was there? What were you

wearing? What were others wearing? What did your sur-
roundings look like? How did you feel? Do you remember
your higher self being there with you at that time?

Take a few moments to continue through the decades of your life, going through one event per decade
that stands out and noticing your higher self in them all.

Now come back to the present moment. Bring your
awareness to challenges you're currently having. Maybe
there is a decision you need to make or a relationship
you need to heal. Whatever it is, ask your witness or
your higher self, "What choice is it in my highest good to
make?" Then scan your body for an inner tug or a sense
of knowing. Your mind will instantly go to a thought
or a solution that hadn't occurred to you before. Your
higher self is now directing your thoughts and helping
you through the power of your intuition.

Your inner witness is always loving, truthful, and
kind. Your higher self will never ask you to do anything or
make any choice that is unloving. If you hear an unloving
voice, that is your ego. When you hear your ego, thank it
and then send it away so you can feel the voice of your
higher self. Continue to do this with every problem you
have, and feel the answer come through your witness.

When you're finished, thank your higher self for its
guidance. You can ask it to help you be more present
with it each day. You can seal your meditation by chanting the mantra sound *SHAM* three times. Take a few
moments before opening your eyes.

You can always come back to this meditation anytime you need to reignite your connection with your
higher self.

ENERGY-BODY HEALING WITH GEMS AND COLORS

Indigo, or bluish-purple, is the color of the sixth chakra. You can wear indigo or adorn a room with this color.

Amethyst, lapis lazuli, and azurite are great stones and crystals to help align the third-eye chakra. Indigo kyanite stimulates the pineal gland and may help awaken psychic abilities.

Sixth Chakra Mindfulness Ideas to Ponder

1. My sense of intuition is as reliable as my senses of sight, smell, hearing, touch, and taste.
2. I will get in touch with my witness or my higher self, and I will practice watching myself in all aspects of life.
3. As I recognize my shadows, they will dissipate, and I will live stronger in the light.
4. Meditation is my path to knowingness and enlightenment.

7 THE CROWN CHAKRA
Sahaswara

COLOR: Violet or White
MANTRA SOUND: *OM*

We have arrived at the top of the seven chakras, the Sahaswara chakra, our source of enlightenment and spiritual connection. This chakra is also referred to as the thousand-petal lotus. In Hindu and Buddhist traditions, the lotus flower is a powerful symbol. It grows through adversity in murky waters and blooms where there is no clarity. The beauty of the lotus emerges out of the darkness. And so it is for you: It has taken you a long time to get here. Your road toward enlightenment has had some bumps and setbacks. Yet here you are, a shining example for the world to see.

The seventh chakra is located at the crown of the head and includes the cerebral cortex, the central nervous system, and the pituitary gland.

Artists have depicted the crown chakra as a halo in paintings and drawings of saints and great spiritual masters. A

Sahaswara person always has a white light glowing around his or her being.

Here a permanent channel is open to divine knowledge and wisdom. The state of seventh chakra awareness exists beyond space, time, and causality. When you attain this state, you merge with oneness. You completely transcend duality. The mind is unaffected by fluctuations and separateness. The seventh chakra person possesses *siddhi* powers, which include clairvoyance, levitation, and psychokinesis.

The Yoga Sutras of Patanjali give us a road map to opening the Sahaswara chakra through the fifth limb of yoga known as pratyahara, or withdrawal of the senses. Through this practice of drawing your senses inward by closing your eyes, observing silence, and minimizing sensory experiences, you access your inner world. Repeated journeys to your inner world create a pathway to enlightenment.

The colors we attribute to the crown chakra are violet and white. No earth elements represent the seventh chakra, as it's a chakra of physical plane transcendence. The mantra, or bija (seed) sound, we vocalize for the seventh chakra is *OM*.

Seventh Chakra Ailments

Diseases and disorders of the seventh chakra include depression, alienation, confusion, boredom, apathy, spiritual skepticism, and inability to learn or comprehend. An out-of-balance crown chakra can also lead to being overly intellectual or feeling spiritually elite or superior.

Seventh Chakra Energy

People who reach seventh chakra energy have achieved what is known in Sanskrit as *guru darshana*. They see and channel messages from the Divine and are able to transmit those messages to others and become dispellers of darkness. They bring enlightenment to others through their wisdom and healing. The energy they receive is pure and unadulterated.

Gurus, or spiritual teachers, who have attained guru darshana have little ego. They have overcome the confines of their egos, so seekers in their presence experience only peace, love, and compassion. The persona we typically extend outward to others with our own ego dissolves in the presence of guru darshana. Therefore seekers can experience spontaneous healing, liberation from past karma, and release when they are with gurus.

The person living in the energy of Sahaswara receives a clear channel of divine knowledge. People living at lower levels of consciousness seek answers from others. They look for other people's opinions and, in some cases, other people's approval. Confusion arises as they keep asking and getting conflicting advice. In the end, they don't know whom to trust or whom to follow. Has this ever happened to you?

You spend a lifetime seeking outside yourself for the answers when the entire time the answers were always inside you. They aren't lurking around your intellect or your ego but rather are in your heart and soul. It's that inner knowing that tells you the right answers.

Naysayers will try to dissuade you. People will tell you you're crazy. But while your choices and answers might be unconventional and sometimes wacky, you will know what is right for you. With confidence you will be able to say to others, "I don't know how I know. I just know."

Our Societal Relationship with the Seventh Chakra

We live in a society of nonbelievers. I understand the boldness in that statement, but it's true. We are a society that wants desperately to believe. Look at all the fantasy movies being produced. Is it any wonder that the Harry Potter series is still one of the bestselling book series today? As a society we want to believe in magic, superpowers, and transcendence. Yet we don't.

If I were to tell you that I have levitated, would you believe me? Well, since you are reading a book on the chakras, you might believe me. However, if I were to tell your brother, sister, mom, dad, or best friend, would they believe me? Probably not. Yet I have. But I don't share that with just anyone, because they either may not take me seriously or they may have me locked up. It is my experience that when you suspend your disbelief long enough to understand that levitation, instant manifestation, or talking to angels is possible, a world of possibilities opens up to you.

I practice and use not only Ayurvedic medicine but also homeopathic medicine. My eldest child, who truly is one of my greatest teachers in patience, said to me with conviction the other day, "You know, homeopathy isn't real. It's just a placebo effect." My eyes opened wide at this statement. "Oh, really," I answered. This same child was healed of many ailments as he grew up on homeopathic medicine. "So," I continued, "you mean to tell me that when homeopathy is used on babies, small children, and animals, it has a placebo effect? They can have no psychophysical response to homeopathy because they're unaware."

My darling child is a single representation of society as a whole. We have abandoned intuition and knowledge of the earth's gifts in pursuit of hard-core scientific fact. If it's not proven, we don't believe it. Yet there is so little we know scientifically. In this great big universe, we've barely scratched the surface.

So what are you to do with seventh chakra awareness as

you live in society? The answer: just be who you are. Once you reach seventh chakra consciousness, you feel no need to prove or defend who you are. Your knowingness transcends any desire to convince or persuade others. Your light is enough to heal others and bring them to you. As for those who aren't ready? You have loving compassion, an understanding for where they are on their journey, and a simple knowingness that the world is perfect as it is.

Living Life in the Sahaswara Chakra

Few people live in the seventh state of consciousness on a daily basis, because doing so requires transcending the ego. The people who have succeeded at this include Jesus, Saint Francis of Assisi, Mother Teresa, Mahatma Gandhi, and Nelson Mandela. I also include Amma, the modern-day saint whom I've had the pleasure of meeting three times and whom I wrote about in the chapter on the Anahata chakra.

My experience with Amma was one that reflects being in the presence of a person who is living in the highest state of consciousness. Two years ago I was waiting to get my hug from Amma. In order to get a hug from her, you must go early in the day and get a number. You then wait your turn to line up. When it's time, you enter a line where you sit in a row of chairs and move up in the chair line until you are next to her. I was about 150 feet from the stage where she was sitting, and I felt an energy I had never before experienced. There was minimal noise in the room, just a low-grade hum of people talking. Spiritual music was playing in the background from a CD, so I knew the vibrations weren't from the music. At that distance from her, my chair was vibrating. It felt as if I were entering a different energy field. To be honest, it was the strangest sensation I have ever felt. From that point forward, as I approached the stage, I stayed in this vibrational frequency, which only got stronger.

Another time I got a hug from Amma, I had a strong but different experience. I didn't feel the vibrations, but as I approached the stage and waited for my hug with just a couple of people ahead of me, I began to spontaneously cry. It wasn't a normal cry but sobs. Moments before, I had felt nothing in particular. I wasn't sad, happy, or stressed. My thoughts weren't on anything in particular. I just started crying. A good friend, who had spent time in Amma's ashram in India, explained that when you are in the presence of a being who is living at seventh chakra consciousness, your energy is cleared just by being near them. Crying was a release, a letting go of negative energy, and some healing occurred.

The power of healing is another ability shared by those living in seventh chakra consciousness. All who live in the energy of Sahaswara have the power to heal. Light emanates from their bodies, and often people are healed just by coming into their presence. Many stories in the Christian scriptures depict Jesus healing the sick, but one story in particular tells of a woman who has a bleeding disorder. She intuitively knows that if she can just touch the cloak of Jesus, she will be healed. And sure enough, when she does, she is indeed healed.

Recognizing Seventh Chakra Imbalances

Imbalances in the seventh chakra can lead to strong limitations. Remember that each chakra has its positive and negative aspects, and the highest chakra is no different. Although you are an unlimited being, you are bound in this life by your physical body and the human experience. And in each stage of spiritual growth, there can be setbacks.

One setback of seventh chakra growth is spiritual elitism. Perhaps you are familiar with the stories in Christian scriptures in which the rabbis and religious elite challenge Jesus on his knowledge of the Hebrew Bible and Jewish doctrine. They try everything they can to stump him. That is a display of spiritual elitism, when people accumulate so much knowledge on spirituality or religion that they deem themselves superior to everyone else. In fact, people who possess this false sense of superiority often act as a replacement for God. Unfortunately, this seems to happen a lot in religious organizations.

In reality, spiritual awareness and connection are much less about knowledge than actual experience. When you experience God, no one can take that away from you. Your knowingness and reality are real. You can be illiterate and still have a seventh chakra awakening.

Please don't take these words as an opportunity to bash religion. I have nothing against organized religion. On the contrary, religion provides a path to higher states of consciousness and spiritual connection. It becomes dangerous only when it claims to take the place of God.

Accepting Seventh Chakra Gifts

Gifts of the seventh chakra are many, and most of us spend our entire lives trying to attain them. Imagine living your life in total peace and bliss. In this space, you are free from worry, anxiety, and sadness. You go through life in total acceptance of the present moment without concern for the future. You live in constant gratitude, awe, and wonder. You are a vessel of unconditional love.

Spiritual literature gives us a road map to acquiring these gifts. In the Christian scriptures, for example, the book of

Matthew, chapters 5 through 7, and the book of John, chapters 14 through 16, tell of all these spiritual gifts and how to attain them. The Yoga Sutras of Patanjali and the wisdom of the Bhagavad Gita can also lead you to a place of peace and surrender. The Tao Te Ching of Taoism and the sacred texts of Buddhism are among others that pave the way toward enlightenment. All these texts give us a step-by-step formula to freely attain seventh chakra gifts. Oh, how foolish we are, those of us who don't take these gifts to heart.

Consider worry, for example. How much time do you waste worrying each day? You worry perhaps about things you can't control such as the weather, the state of the world, or the way people around you are acting. Then you probably spend time worrying about things you can control but for which you can't control the outcome. For example, I know people who worry constantly about losing their job. You can control getting to work on time, doing extraordinary work, and being a good team player. But you can't control the potential outcome of your company needing to downsize. When things are not going according to your expectations, you worry. When things are going well, you worry that they might turn bad. All in all, worry steals you from your life and your bliss.

Yet all the spiritual masters and all the spiritual literature tell you not to worry. Jesus himself spent three years in his ministry, and we only have a limited amount of direct teaching in his words, through the Christian Gospels. So you know that if Jesus taught something and said it more than once, it must be pretty important. In the book of Matthew, chapter 6, Jesus spends no less than ten verses talking about how we shouldn't worry. In verse 25 he says, "That is why I tell you not to worry about everyday life," and he concludes with verse 34: "So don't worry about tomorrow, for tomorrow will bring its own worries. Today's trouble is enough for today."

Other spiritual masters speak about living in the present moment. Yoga and meditation teach us present-moment awareness. Worry is living in the past or in the future but not in the present. Worry is a thief who comes to steal your joy and peace. Just as you would never welcome a robber into your home to take your things, why welcome worry into your mind?

By the time you have awakened to the seventh chakra, your understanding of oneness with universal consciousness doesn't even allow you to entertain emotions such as worry. For if you are one with the universe, there is no lack and therefore no worry. But I hope my example has provided you with a vision of where you are today in comparison to where you would like to be. And whenever you need a reminder, spiritual literature is there to point the way to the peace of the seventh chakra.

Healing Sahaswara

DAILY AFFIRMATION
I am one with the Divine.

 ### Healing the Physical Body

Besides the practice of meditation, which we discussed in relation to the sixth chakra, getting into the seventh chakra zone is best achieved through the practices of silence, reading spiritual and inspirational literature, and spending time in nature. Sometimes we spontaneously connect with the Divine in moments when we don't expect it, but most of the time it happens because we make a conscious effort to create an environment in which connection can happen. That is why people often feel connected to the Divine when they go to a church or synagogue but then feel disconnected for the rest of the week. As you have seen, the road to spirituality requires effort.

What you move toward expands, and what you move away from diminishes. For example, if your focus is on your work, often your home life suffers. When your focus is on your relationships, your work may suffer. The same goes for your spiritual life: when you place your focus there, your connection to the Divine will grow, while other, less-important areas will fade into the background.

The other day I was in the car with my twenty-two-year-old, who after fifteen minutes or so turned on the radio and said, "I hate it that you drive around in silence. What's wrong with you? It's very disturbing." I hadn't even noticed. I love silence. I've been practicing silence in everything I do for years. On most occasions I keep the radio and TV off. While I love music, I rarely listen to it now. I just love silence. I love listening to the noises in the environment: the birds, the crickets, and even the cars passing by. Silence is a profound gift, and I believe it's God's one and only true voice. When you reach the seventh chakra level of consciousness, you're no longer afraid of your mind and your thoughts. I have noticed that fear of silence is fear of one's own mind. Your mind is your friend, not your enemy. The more you believe that, the more you can sit in silence and not only be comfortable in it but even crave more of it.

Spend time reading spiritual literature, whether it's poetry or scripture. Immerse yourself in nature whenever you can to enjoy everything that connects you to the heartbeat of the universe.

Yoga Asanas and Pranayama Exercises to Heal the Seventh Chakra

Try these breathing techniques and poses to help open and align the Sahaswara chakra.

To view a video demo of these exercises, go to
www.youtube.com/c/MichelleFondinAuthor.
Click on the Playlists tab, and select
Chakra Healing Asanas & Pranayamas.
Scroll down the list until you find the one you're looking for.

Skull Shining Breath — *Kapalabhati*: Kapalabhati is done by inhaling passively and exhaling forcefully, both through the nose. Exhaling in this way contracts the lower abdominal muscles, so you may feel as if you have done a lot of sit-ups after doing this breathing technique.

Sit with your spine tall, and close your eyes. Inhale deeply through your nose, and then exhale completely. Inhale passively through the nose, then exhale forcefully. Continue with this pattern for about one minute. When you finish, take a deep breath in, and then exhale completely.

Wide-Angle Standing Forward Fold — *Prasarita Padottanasana*: For this pose, stand on a yoga mat and have a couple of yoga blocks or a chair in front of you. Stand with your feet one leg length's distance apart with your toes pointing forward. Lift your torso tall and bend forward from your hips, bringing your hands to the floor. If you have a difficult time bringing your head close to the floor, bring your feet a little wider apart. Bend your elbows and bring the crown of your head toward the floor. To assist you, you can either place your head on top of the yoga blocks or on the chair seat. Stay in the forward fold for at least five breaths. To come up, bend at your knees and gently roll up to standing.

Fish Pose — *Matsyasana*: Lying on your mat, bend both knees with your feet flat on the floor. Lift your hips, bring your arms underneath your buttocks with your palms pressing into the floor, and lower your hips back down to the mat so you're sitting on your hands. Straighten your legs on the floor, and bring your feet together so your big toes touch. Press down on your elbows and forearms, and lift your chest and head. Tilt your head back, and place the crown of your head on the floor. Hold for five breaths. To get out of the pose, press down on your elbows and lift your head off the floor. Bring your head gently down into alignment with your spine, and release your arms. As a counterpose, lie in *savasana*, or relaxation pose, for about five even, slow breaths before moving on to the next pose.

Headstand — *Salamba Sirsasana*: This pose is for advanced yoga students only. If you're new to doing headstands, it's best to use a wall as a support. Bring your mat to the wall. Begin the pose on your hands and knees about five inches away from the wall. Come down to your elbows, and fold your hands in front of you. Your folded hands and elbows will form a triangle. Make sure your elbows are directly underneath your shoulders. Lock your shoulders and shoulder blades back toward your spine to have a strong support. Open the palms of your folded hands and bring your thumbs straight up. You're forming a cup for your head. Place the top of your head on the floor, with the back of your head in your cupped hands. Lift your pelvis in the air so you're standing on your tiptoes, as in the dolphin pose. Your body will look like an upside-down letter *V*. Walk your feet toward your elbows. When you feel ready, lift your legs straight up and toward the wall. You might want to do one leg at a time. You can rest your legs on the wall and then readjust your posture to maintain the pose. Stay for up to three minutes. As you hold your headstand, the crown of your head will barely touch the floor. To come down, gently lower one leg at a time. Go into child's pose (balasana) as a counterpose: lower your hips to the floor, and then extend your torso forward and rest it between your thighs, with your forehead on the floor.

 ## Healing the Emotional and Energetic Body

By the time you arrive at the seventh chakra, you have worked through blockages in your emotional body and have brought awareness to your shadows. Through your practice of meditation, you will experience increasingly frequent peak states and moments of bliss.

Peak States

Chances are, you have had moments in your life when everything seemed perfect. In these moments you were on top of the world. Life flowed, and you knew that nothing could go wrong. You may have been taking care of your baby, making love, or working on a passion project. Maybe you were just walking in nature or observing a sunset, and time stood still while you experienced wonder and awe.

Peak states are when you transcend space and time. At first, these moments seem to come out of nowhere. They're amazingly perfect, and you don't want them to end. But when you try to grasp them or make them occur again, they don't come when you want. For example, you go hiking and have a marvelous feeling of connectedness, and then you tell a friend about it, urging her to join you the next time. Yet the next time isn't quite as magical, and you're disappointed because you really wanted her to experience the same feeling you had. That is generally how peak states work. They happen when you merge into oneness through surrender, but you can't necessarily replicate them. The more you practice meditation and accept the seventh chakra's spiritual gifts, however, the more readily you will experience peak states.

BLISS

I describe bliss as an extended peak state. In peak states, you experience bliss. But because of the turmoil of the mind, as soon as you realize you're in bliss your mind comes in and gives you reasons why you shouldn't be, and the peak state ends. That pesky mind of yours (and mine) can be a big buzzkill.

Bliss is not happiness. Happiness is a transitory state that is based on external factors such as people, places, or things. Bliss comes from a place that is internal. It comes when you repeatedly turn inward through meditation, and over time you will find that you can remain there for extended periods. Once you attain bliss, it can't be taken away from you. Your bliss comes from oneness with God and divine unconditional love.

 Healing the Spiritual Body

Yogastah, kuru karmani.
Established in being, perform action.
— BHAGAVAD GITA 2:48

ESTABLISHED IN BEING

Most people search their whole lives for a solid spiritual connection but never attain it. Remember the song lyric "Looking for love in all the wrong places"? Many look for enlightenment in all the wrong places, such as in material items, experiences, and other people. They are constantly searching the world outside themselves for the answers, when the answers they seek are inside.

When you finally come to an understanding that your spiritual connection is here — that it never left you and that you can experience it now — you may crave it all the time. It can be all too easy to want to stay in bliss and joy. So you want to do yoga five days a week, spend hours daily in meditation, and attend as many spiritual gatherings as you can for fear that this connection might leave you. As a former yoga studio owner, I have seen yoga students search for bliss in the same way they might search for a buzz from alcohol. They need it and feel that they "gotta have it."

True peace comes from a seventh chakra awakening that you don't need to chase something that is ever present. Your peace, joy, and bliss are there when you wake up, eat breakfast, do the dishes, dress your kids, go grocery shopping, drive, and do thousands of other things as you go about your day.

In the Hindu spiritual text the Bhagavad Gita, which means the "Song of the Lord," Arjuna, a warrior, has a conversation with his charioteer, Krishna, who is God incarnate. Arjuna is worried about many things and does not want to perform his duty out of fear. Krishna helps Arjuna see that as long as he is connected to God, he can let go and perform action. It comes from the realization that he, Arjuna, is not in charge of what happens; God is.

When you're aware that you are tethered to God, your actions, whatever the outcome, are divinely guided. But you have to let go of fear and plunge into your daily activities.

B. K. S. Iyengar, one of the greatest yogis of our modern age, was a householder. He had a wife and kids. He explains that staying true to your duties as a husband, provider, and father is enlightenment. As an enlightened being, you're no good to the world if you stay hidden in a cave or an enclosed room, living alone and meditating all day. Part of living an enlightened life is going out there, established in being — meaning connected to God and your higher self — and actually living.

The great sages and saints of all time, from whom we have learned, did this. For example, Jesus of Nazareth spent three years of his life, leading up to his death, facing all kinds of adversity. He didn't say, "I'm just going to stay over here and pray to my Father and meditate. Apostles, you guys go out and preach for me." He went out there and healed the sick, talked about God to people who thought he was not only crazy but also an imposter, and inspired thousands with his words, all while people were plotting to kill him. Talk about taking action!

Another aspect of living life established in being is authenticity — in other words, being yourself. You are not Mahatma Gandhi or Mother Teresa, nor could you be them if you tried. Even in enlightenment, you are still you. You have your personality, your unique gifts and talents, and your flaws. Many seekers try to be just like the spiritual masters they love. But, of course, when they try to be someone else, they invariably fall short. They're left wearing a mask, and they become unauthentic.

Since I'm a yoga and meditation teacher, I meet all types of people. Some people in New Age circles try to be perfect spiritual beings. They speak their own language, always talking about the chakras and saying words in Sanskrit. That's well and good, but there can be a disingenuous air to it all. I've seen the same thing in Christian circles too. Just because you understand spiritual truths doesn't mean you must act a certain way and use a different vocabulary. In fact, when you really understand spiritual truths, you become even more down-to-earth. You're even more in touch with what it means to be human. You can relate better to humanness. When you perform action, you're a conduit for God's work.

COCREATING WITH GOD

Miracles occur at the seventh chakra level of consciousness, as you have an inner knowing that you are a cocreator with God. When you are established in being, you seek to do God's will in all things. Therefore your desires become God's desires. As such, you become a powerful manifestor. You then experience spontaneous fulfillment of desire. Whatever you place your attention on becomes real in material form. Your life becomes magical each and every day. The struggles you experience aren't struggles at all; they're only God's way of redirecting you into the path God has chosen for you. You see beauty in all and through all. Opportunities await you at every step. Your daily mantra shifts from "What's in it for me?" to "How can I help? How can I serve? How can I do your will, God?" Your needs are automatically taken care of as you fully live your life's purpose. Bliss is your permanent state.

SAHASWARA GUIDED MEDITATION

Sit or lie comfortably and close your eyes. Take in a full belly breath, and exhale completely. Repeat the full breath seven times to feel the energy of each chakra rising upward toward the seventh. Now place your awareness on the top of your head, the crown chakra. Imagine a beautiful violet thousand-petal lotus flower sitting there and bringing you its wisdom. Next, imagine a flood of white light pouring down upon you from the heavens, coming in through the crown of your head and then infiltrating your whole body. See this white light filling every one of your cells. The boundaries in your body dissolve as the light fills every gap and space in your physical body. The light is so bright and intense that you feel it radiating from the inside out. Even with your eyes still closed you can feel and see light radiating from your fingers and toes, from your arms and legs, and then from the rest of your body. Feel this fast vibration of light pulsating through you. You may even feel your body rocking, and that is okay. Go with it as you feel this powerful force of light.

Now bring to your attention any ascended masters who resonate with you. Ascended masters are those divine beings who walked the earth and became great spiritual teachers. You can call to Jesus, Moses, Mother Mary, the Prophet Muhammad, Paramahansa Yogananda, Mother Teresa, Siddhartha Gautama Buddha, or any other ascended master who inspires you. Call to the great spiritual leaders and ask them to guide you in the highest light and love of God. Ask that they show you the way to the highest vibrational frequency of seventh chakra awareness. Listen to any messages they might have for you now. You will hear these messages as a sudden thought, intuition, or hunch. Sit in the peaceful presence of these divine masters. When you are finished, thank them for their peace and guidance.

Feel the essence of being merged with the One. You

are boundless. You are whole. You are one with the Divine. You are infinite perfection and infinite intelligence. You know now that all thoughts of separateness are an illusion. When you come out of this meditation, you will continue to remember. You will continue to feel connected. You will remain established in being.

Rest in this state of perfection for as long as you choose. When it is time to return to activity, conclude your meditation by chanting *OM* seven times.

ENERGY-BODY HEALING WITH GEMS AND COLORS

The colors of the Sahaswara chakra are violet and white. Wearing these colors and surrounding yourself with them will help remind you of seventh chakra energy.

Two gemstones for the seventh chakra are amethyst and diamond.

Seventh Chakra Mindfulness Ideas to Ponder

1. I fully and openly accept all the spiritual gifts offered to me today.
2. I totally immerse myself in present-moment awareness.
3. I hold in my mind the great spiritual masters who continue to influence my life, and I ask them to stay with me throughout my day.
4. I am one with the Divine. I remain in the state of infinite perfection.

CONCLUSION
Maximize Your Healing Power

On your chakra healing journey, remember to have faith that you can heal. Your body is an amazing healing machine that is designed for perfect health. However, you have been raised in a family, social system, and society with certain beliefs about health and healing, including skepticism of nontraditional modalities. Chances are you have unconsciously adopted limiting thoughts about what is possible, and this type of social conditioning is not easy to overcome. Perhaps you can understand and feel the possibilities of energy healing, yet at times living in this world of disbelief weighs heavily on your newfound freedom. The solution: just keep practicing.

In chakra healing, as in anything you'd like to get good at, you need practice. Practice adopting these principles. Reread each chapter thoroughly. You may need to put yourself on a program to gradually change your mind-set. As mentioned in the beginning of the book, you can take seven days to begin healing your chakras with one chakra for each day. Or you can take one chakra per week or per month. Each time you repeat the exercises for a given chakra, your healing and understanding will deepen. Gradual awakening will take place as you uncover the layers of your existence.

Be Patient with Your Healing Process

Remember how long it has taken you to get to this point in your life. You may have spent twenty, thirty, forty, fifty years or more thinking and behaving in a certain way. Disease is not formed overnight. Imbalances are created over time. Likewise, healing them takes time. Also, keep in mind that the feeling of wellness often precedes improvement of physical symptoms. Have you ever had a cold or flu and started to feel better in your mind and noticed that your body was starting to heal, but your nose was still running like crazy? That's because physical matter takes time to catch up. Stay the course, and even though you can't see anything in the physical world, know that changes are taking place within you.

Be Patient with Others

As you begin to see life with a wider perception, you may notice that other people in your immediate circle are not on the same spiritual path. Not only is this realization difficult, but it can also be downright frustrating. At those moments, it's important to remember that each person has his or her own path and life purpose. It's counterproductive to try to drag a loved one off his or her path and onto yours. The best way you can help others is to show by example. When you attain greater peace, compassion, and love, you attract others to your path. Even if your spouse, best friend, or child never joins you on your path, the relationship will change as you reach higher states of awareness.

Adopt a Lifetime of Healing

The practices outlined and suggested in this book are designed for you to adopt for a lifetime. There may have been a time in your life when you started a new practice such as yoga, meditation, healthy eating, or exercise, and you began to see results. But for some reason, you stopped, went back to your old ways, and started to feel bad again. To experience a lifetime of health, allow yourself enough time to not only feel fantastic but also adopt each practice as a habit.

When I started my meditation practice in November 2007, I meditated every day. I kept at it faithfully for months. I trained my brain, mind, and body to expect meditation and to need it. After a few months my body began to crave meditation. If I didn't do it, I felt terrible. You want your body to have this type of response. You want to fill it with many good, healthy practices so that when you don't do them, you crave them. Then and only then will you know that you've made permanent and lasting changes.

Know That I Am with You

I'm with you on your healing journey, and so are all the other people who have accepted this healing path. You can draw from our energy when you're feeling weak or that something isn't working. We meet in the infinite field when meditating. Our energy extends outward to you. Remain open to receiving. Stay strong, flexible, and rooted. Your light is needed so we can reach critical mass and raise the consciousness of the world. Love and light to you always. *Om shanti, shanti, shanti.* Namasté.

ACKNOWLEDGMENTS

My heartfelt gratitude goes to Georgia Hughes, New World Library's editorial director. You took a huge leap of faith with an indie author after meeting me at Book Expo America in 2014, and now we're on our second book together. Thank you for believing in me.

A big thank-you goes to Kristen Cashman and Emily Wichland for patiently and graciously editing my work.

Thank you to New World Library publicists Kim Corbin, Monique Muhlenkamp, and Tristy Taylor for lining me up with great interviews, reviews, and press.

A big shout-out goes to Foreign Rights Manager Danielle Galat. We did it for *The Wheel of Healing with Ayurveda* — five languages and counting — and here's to getting even more translations this time.

And finally, thank you to Marc Allen for founding and running such a great publishing firm. It's hard for a new author to know all the work that goes into publishing a single title, and New World Library does a great job of it.

GLOSSARY OF SANSKRIT TERMS

ABHYANGA: Daily oil massage.

AGNI: Fire; in Ayurveda, digestive fire.

AJNA: The sixth chakra; *Ajna* translates as "to perceive or command" or "beyond wisdom."

AKASHA: Space or ether.

AMA: A toxic residue caused by undigested food, experiences, and emotions. The term translates as "toxins in the body and mind."

ANAHATA: The fourth chakra; *Anahata* translates as "unstruck" or "unhurt."

ARTHA: Material wealth, gain, or prosperity. One of the four goals in life that are known, in Vedic morality, as the *purusharthas.*

ASANA: Physical postures; the third limb of yoga.

AYURVEDA: The science of life; the name is derived from the Sanskrit words *ayus*, meaning "life," and *veda*, meaning "science or knowledge."

BANDHA: Bond or arrest; in Hatha yoga, translated as "body locks."

BIJA: Seed; or the seed syllable contained within a mantra.

BRAMACHARYA: Celibacy or sexual restraint; the fourth of the yamas in the Yoga Sutras of Patanjali.

CHAKRAS: The energy centers in the body. There are seven main chakras from the base of the spine to the crown of the head.

DHARANA: One-pointed attention or fixed concentration on something internal or external; the sixth limb of yoga.

DHARMA: An individual's purpose in life.

DHYANA: Meditation; the seventh limb of yoga.

DIRGHA: Also called the three-part or complete breath, a yogic breathing exercise that trains the body to breathe from the diaphragm.

DOSHA: The three main psychophysiological principles of the body (Vata, Pitta, Kapha), which determine a person's individual mind-body constitution.

DRISHTI: To view or gaze; in relation to yoga, it means "focal point."

GHEE: Clarified butter.

GUNAS: The three fundamental forces or qualities of nature: sattva, rajas, and tamas.

GURU DARSHANA: Auspicious sight given to a devotee by an enlightened teacher (guru).

IDA NADI: The left subtle channel, which is feminine and lunar in nature.

JALA: Water.

KAPHA: One of the three doshas, it combines the elements water and earth. It is responsible for bodily structure.

KARMA: Action or deed. It is also the principle of causality, in which a person's intent in taking an action in the present equals a particular result in the future.

KUNDALINI: Divine female energy that lies latent at the base of the spine.

KUNDALINI SHAKTI: The awakening of Kundalini as it uncoils and makes its way up the spine toward Shiva (male) energy.

MAHABHUTAS: The great elements: space, air, fire, water, and earth.

MANIPURA: The third chakra; *Manipura* translates as "lustrous gem."

MANTRA: Derived from two Sanskrit words: *man*, meaning "mind," and *tra*, meaning "instrument." This instrument of the mind is a sound or series of sounds used to connect body, mind, and spirit.

MOKSHA: Liberation or freedom.

MULADHARA: The first chakra; *Muladhara* translates as "root" or "support."

NADI: A subtle circulatory channel running through the body that carries energy and information. The three main nadis are Ida, Pingala, and Shushumna.

NASYA: Method of administering oil or herbalized oil to the nostrils. It is one of the five parts of *panchakarma*.

NIYAMAS: Internal observances or duties; the second limb of yoga.

OJAS: Healing chemicals in the body that are by-products of properly digested food, emotions, and experiences.

PANCHAKARMA: "Five Actions"; a program of detoxification of the body in Ayurvedic medicine.

PINGALA NADI: The right subtle channel, which is masculine and solar in nature.

PITTA: The dosha in Ayurveda composed of the elements fire and water.

PRAKRUTI: Physical matter; also, the biological constitution of an individual, determined at conception and composed of certain proportions of the three doshas: Vata, Pitta, and Kapha.

PRANA: Vital life energy, or life force.

PRANA VATA: One of the five subdoshas of Vata in Ayurveda;

controls inhalation, consumption, perception, and the intake of knowledge.

PRANAYAMA: Yogic breathing techniques; the fourth limb of yoga.

PRATYAHARA: Withdrawal of the senses; the fifth limb of yoga.

PRITHIVI: The earth element.

PURUSHA: The cosmic Self (soul), cosmic consciousness, or the universal principle; unbounded universal energy that has not yet taken form into *prakruti*.

RAJAS: Activity, energy, passion, restlessness; one of the three primary qualities of nature in yoga philosophy.

RISHIS: Ancient sages, or seers, from India.

SAHASWARA: The seventh chakra; *Sahaswara* translates as "thousand-petal lotus."

SAMADHI: An advanced state of meditation, marked by oneness or absorption of the self; the eighth limb of yoga.

SATTVA: Purity, one of the three primary qualities of nature in yoga philosophy.

SHAKTI: Energy, power, movement, or change; the female principle of divine energy, especially in mythology when referring to a deity.

SHUKRA: Lucid, clear, bright.

SHUKRA DHATU: In Ayurvedic medicine, reproductive tissue in both men and women.

SHUSHUMNA: The central nadi in the body aligning along the spine; translates as "very gracious" or "kind."

SIDDHI: Supernatural power; realization, attainment.

SUBDOSHAS: The five subdivisions of each of the three doshas in Ayurveda with physiological structures in the human body.

SURYA NAMASKAR: Sun Salutations, a series of yoga poses that coordinates with the breath.

SVADHISTHANA: The second chakra; *Svadhisthana* translates as "the dwelling place of the self."

TAMAS: Inertia, lethargy, darkness, or dullness, one of the three primary qualities of nature in yoga philosophy.

TANMANTRAS: Subtle elements. In Ayurveda, refers to the five senses: hearing, touch, taste, sight, and smell.

TANTRA: An ancient set of esoteric texts originally from Hindu or Buddhist tradition dating from the sixth to the thirteenth centuries of the common era; translated as "to weave."

TEJAS: Fire.

TRIPHALA: A rejuvenating herbal remedy in Ayurvedic medicine composed of three herbs: amalaki, bibitaki, and haritaki.

VATA: Composed of space and air, one of the three doshas, or Ayurvedic mind-body types.

VAYU: Wind or air.

VISHUDDHA: The fifth chakra; *Vishuddha* translates as "purity."

YAMAS: Moral, ethical, and social guidelines for the practicing yogi; the first limb of yoga, outlined in the first of the Yoga Sutras of Patanjali.

YOGA: Derived from the Sanskrit word *yuj,* which means "to yoke" or "to join together." In yoga, we join together our mind, body, soul, and spirit.

YOGA SUTRAS OF PATANJALI: The basic philosophical writings of yoga, compiled around 400 CE, containing four chapters or books separated into 196 sutras, or aphorisms. It outlines the eight limbs of yoga: yama, niyama, asana, pranayama, pratyahara, dharana, dhyana, samadhi.

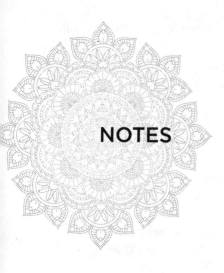

NOTES

Introduction

Page 5, *"and breathed into his nostrils the breath of life"*: Genesis 2:7, New International Version.

1. The Root Chakra

Page 26, *"We should have a liver appreciation day"*: Wayne W. Dyer, *The Awakened Life*, audio CD set, Simon & Schuster Audio/Nightingale-Conant, 2006.

Page 30, *Can all your worries*: Matthew 6:27, New Living Translation.

2. The Sacral Chakra

Page 43, *Chronic lifestyle diseases such as diabetes*: Partnership to Fight Chronic Disease, "The Growing Crisis of Chronic Disease in the United States," https://www.fightchronicdisease.org/sites/default/files

/docs/GrowingCrisisofChronicDiseaseintheUSfactsheet_81009.pdf, accessed November 30, 2017.

Page 49, *He calls this power sex transmutation*: Napoleon Hill, *Think and Grow Rich* (New York: Fawcett Books, 1960), 175–96.

Page 58, *the January 11, 2017, issue of* The Lancet: Harvard Health Publishing, Harvard Medical School, "Uncovering the Link between Emotional Stress and Heart Disease," April 2017, https://www.health.harvard.edu/heart-disease-overview/uncovering-the-link-between-emotional-stress-and-heart-disease.

Page 61, *"The great artists, writers, musicians, and poets become great"*: Hill, *Think and Grow Rich*, 179.

Page 62, *"Everything in your external world"*: Anthony Robbins, *Get the Edge: A 7-Day Program to Transform Your Life*, 10-CD set, 2001.

4. The Heart Chakra

Page 91, *In the United States, heart disease is*: Centers for Disease Control and Prevention, "Health, United States 2016: With Chartbook on Long-Term Trends in Health," May 2017, https://www.cdc.gov/nchs/data/hus/hus16.pdf#019. Also, Centers for Disease Control and Prevention, "Leading Causes of Death," March 17, 2017, https://www.cdc.gov/nchs/fastats/leading-causes-of-death.htm.

Page 92, *"Father, forgive them, for they know not what they do"*: Luke 23:34, English Standard Version.

Page 92, *Hurricane Harvey damaged 203,000 homes*: Kimberly Amadeo, "Hurricane Harvey Facts, Damage, and Costs," *The Balance*, September 30, 2017, https://www.thebalance.com/hurricane-harvey-facts-damage-costs-4150087.

Page 92, *American companies pledged over $157 million*: Kaya Yurieff, "Businesses Donate Over $157 Million to Harvey Relief Efforts," CNN Money, September 3, 2017, http://money.cnn.com/2017/08/30/news/companies/hurricane-harvey-corporate-donations/index.html.

Page 95, *As Pope Francis so eloquently voiced*: Angela Dewan, "Pope Warns against Walls ahead of US Election," CNN, November 7, 2016, http://www.cnn.com/2016/11/06/europe/pope-walls-us-election-trump/index.html.

Page 96, *"If it is one man's karma to suffer"*: "About Amma Amritananda-mayi: How She Began," Amma.org, http://amma.org/about/how-she -began, accessed November 15, 2017.

Page 98, *"Where is the enjoyment in chaos and hysteria?"*: Deepak Chopra, *Primordial Sound Meditation Course on the 7 States of Consciousness,* DVD.

Page 98, *This great organization has managed to*: "History: Saving Lives, Serving People," MADD, https://www.madd.org/history, accessed December 1, 2017.

Page 107, *"I can choose peace rather than this"*: Mary NurrieStearns, "Manifesting Spiritual Change: An Interview with Wayne Dyer," Personal Transformation, http://www.personaltransformation.com /wayne_dyer.html, accessed November 15, 2017.

Page 108, *"Love is always open arms"*: Leo Buscaglia, *Love: What Life Is About* (New York: Fawcett Books, 1972), 64.

6. The Third-Eye Chakra

Page 142, *"Ajna is where time ceases to exist"*: Dr. K.O. Paulose, "Agnya Chakra or Third Eye Chakra," May 10, 2010, http://drpaulose.com /general/agnya-chakra-or-third-eye-chakra.

Page 146, *According to the Centers for Disease Control*: "Chronic Diseases: The Leading Causes of Death and Disability in the United States," Centers for Disease Control and Prevention, https://www.cdc.gov /chronicdisease/overview/index.htm, accessed December 1, 2017.

Page 152, *According to a Mayo Clinic article*: "Seasonal Affective Dis-order Treatment: Choosing a Light Therapy Box," Mayo Clinic, https://www.mayoclinic.org/diseases-conditions/seasonal-affective -disorder/in-depth/seasonal-affective-disorder-treatment/art-2004 8298?pg=2, accessed December 1, 2017.

Page 159, *Dr. Wayne W. Dyer used to say*: Dr. Wayne W. Dyer, *Your Sacred Self: Making the Decision to Be Free* (New York: HarperCollins, 1995).

7. The Crown Chakra

Page 170, *"That is why I tell you not to worry"*: Matthew 6:25 and Matthew 6:34, New Living Translation.

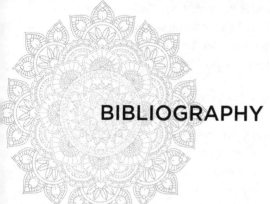

BIBLIOGRAPHY

Bailey, James. "Discover the Ida and Pingala Nadis." *Yoga Journal*. August 28, 2007. http://www.yogajournal.com/yoga-101/balancing-act-2.

Burgin, Timothy. "The 3 Gunas of Nature." Yoga Basics. http://www.yoga basics.com/learn/the-3-gunas-of-nature/.

Burton, Neel. "These Are the Seven Types of Love: And How We Can Ignore the Most Available and Potentially Fulfilling Types." *Psychology Today*. June 25, 2016. https://www.psychologytoday.com/blog/hide -and-seek/201606/these-are-the-7-types-love.

"Chronic Diseases: The Leading Causes of Death and Disability in the United States." Centers for Disease Control and Prevention. Last modified February 23, 2016, https://www.cdc.gov/chronicdisease/overview/.

Feldsher, Karen. "Take It to Heart: Positive Emotions May Be Good for Health." Harvard T. H. Chan School of Public Health. https://www .hsph.harvard.edu/news/features/positive-emotions-health -kubzansky-html/.

Frawley, David. "The Purusha Principle of Yoga." Excerpt from *Yoga and the Sacred Fire*. American Institute of Vedic Studies. June 13, 2012. https://vedanet.com/2012/06/13/the-purusha-principle-of-yoga.

Hartranft, Chip. *The Yoga-Sutra of Patanjali: A New Translation with Commentary*. Boston: Shambhala Publications, 2003.

Hill, Napoleon. *Think and Grow Rich*. New York: Fawcett Books, 1937.

Johari, Harish. *Chakras: Energy Centers of Transformation*. Rochester, VT: Destiny Books, 2000.

Judith, Anodea. *Wheels of Life: A User's Guide to the Chakra System*. St. Paul, MN: Llewellyn Publications, 1994.

Krznaric, Roman. "The Ancient Greeks' Six Words for Love (and Why Knowing Them Can Change Your Life)." *Yes!* magazine. December 27, 2013. http://www.yesmagazine.org/happiness/the-ancient-greeks-6-words-for-love-and-why-knowing-them-can-change-your-life.

Lad, Vasant. *Textbook of Ayurveda*. Vol. 3, *General Principles of Management and Treatment*. Albuquerque, NM: Ayurvedic Press, 325–27.

Le Page, Lillian, and Joseph Le Page. *Yoga Toolbox for Teachers and Students: Yoga Posture Cards for Integrating Mind, Body & Spirit*. Santa Rosa, CA: Integrative Yoga Therapy, 2005.

New Believer's Bible: First Steps for New Christians. New Living Translation. Carol Stream, IL: Tyndale House Publishers, 1996, 2006.

Radin, Dean. "Attaining the Siddhis: Twenty-Five Superhuman Powers You Can Gain through Practicing Yoga and Meditation." *Conscience Lifestyle* magazine. http://www.consciouslifestylemag.com/siddhis-attain-yoga-powers/.

Ram, Bhava. *The 8 Limbs of Yoga: Pathway to Liberation*. Coronado, CA: Deep Yoga, 2009.

Swami Jnaneshvara. "Yoga Sutras 4.13–4.14: Objects and the Three Gunas." Swamij.com. http://www.swamij.com/yoga-sutras-41314.htm.

Venusia, Anjani. "The 3 Gunas: Satva, Rajas, Tamas." http://initiate ayurveda.blogspot.com/p/3-gunas-satva-rajas-tamas.html.

INDEX OF YOGA ASANAS AND PRANAYAMA PRACTICES

INDEX OF AILMENTS
RELATED TO THE CHAKRAS

ABOUT THE AUTHOR

Michelle S. Fondin is the owner of Fondin Wellness, where she practices as an Ayurvedic lifestyle counselor and as a yoga and meditation teacher. She holds a Vedic Master certificate from the Chopra Center and has worked with Dr. Deepak Chopra at Chopra Center events teaching yoga and meditation. Her new passion is creating videos for YouTube, and she has found that it not only allows her to help viewers, but satisfies her taste for being in front of the camera. When Michelle isn't writing, teaching, or filming, she likes to travel, spend time with her teenage children, run half-marathons, and go salsa dancing.

Subscribe to Michelle's YouTube channel to see videos on health and wellness:

www.youtube.com/c/MichelleFondinAuthor

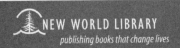